COLLABORATIVE PRACTICE IN PALLIATIVE CARE

Collaborative Practice in Palliative Care explores how different professions work collaboratively across professional, institutional, social, and cultural boundaries to enhance palliative care.

Analysing palliative care as an interaction between different professionals, clients, and carers, and the social context or community within which the interaction takes place, it is grounded in up-to-date evidence, includes global aspects of palliative care and cultural diversity as themes running throughout the book, and is replete with examples of good and innovative practice. Drawing on experiences from within traditional specialist palliative care settings like hospices and community palliative care services, as well as more generalist contexts of the general hospital and primary care, this practical text highlights the social or public health model of palliative care. Designed to support active learning, it includes features such as case studies, summaries, and pointers to other learning resources.

This text is an important reference for all professionals engaged in palliative care, particularly those studying for post-qualification programmes in the area.

Dave Roberts is Senior Lecturer in Cancer and Palliative Care at Oxford Brookes University. His research interests and publications focus primarily on psychosocial aspects of health, principally cancer & palliative care, communication skills, and psychological interventions, and global aspects of health care and education.

Laura Green is Lecturer in Adult Nursing at the University of Manchester, teaching palliative and end of life care at pre-registration and Masters level programmes. She is Deputy Director of the Non-Medical Prescribing Programme. She is a member of the University's Research Ethics Panel. Her clinical experience is as a Clinical Nurse Specialist in Palliative Care, and a nurse working in the community and hospice settings. Laura is one of three nurses who established @WeEOLC, an online Twitter community of learning and practice, and is a regular host of Tweet Chats. She blogs at www.lmiddletongreen.wordpress.com and tweets as @heblau and @WeEOLC.

CAIPE Collaborative Practice Series

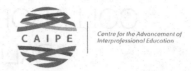

Centre for the Advancement of
Interprofessional Education

Founded in 1987, CAIPE is a charity and company limited by guarantee which promotes and develops interprofessional education with and through its members. It works with like-minded organisations in the UK and overseas to improve collaborative practice, patient safety and quality of care by professions learning and working together. CAIPE's contributions to IPE include publications, development workshops, consultancy, commissioned studies and international partnerships, projects and networks.

CAIPE not only offers expertise and experience, but also provides an independent perspective which can facilitate collaboration across the boundaries between education and health, health and social care, and beyond. Membership of CAIPE is open to individuals, students and organisations such as academic institutions, independent and public service providers in the UK and overseas. For further information about CAIPE and other benefits of membership go to www.caipe.org.uk

Series Editors:
Hugh Barr
Marion Helme
Maggie Hutchings, Bournemouth University, UK
Alison Machin, Northumbria University, UK

Published titles:

Collaborative Practice with Vulnerable Children and their Families
Julie Taylor, June Thoburn

Collaborative Practice for Public Health
Dawne Gurbutt

Collaborative Practice in Critical Care Settings
A Workbook
Scott Reeves, Janet Alexanian, Deborah Kendall-Gallagher, Todd Dorman and Simon Kitto

Collaborative Practice in Primary and Community Care
Edited by Sanjiv Ahluwalia, John Spicer and Karen Storey

Collaborative Practice in Palliative Care
Edited by Dave Roberts and Laura Green

For more information about this series, please visit: https://www.routledge.com/CAIPE-Collaborative-Practice-Series/book-series/CAIPE

Collaborative Practice in Palliative Care

Edited by
Dave Roberts
and Laura Green

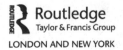

Routledge
Taylor & Francis Group

LONDON AND NEW YORK

First published 2022
by Routledge
2 Park Square, Milton Park, Abingdon, Oxon OX14 4RN

and by Routledge
605 Third Avenue, New York, NY 10158

Routledge is an imprint of the Taylor & Francis Group, an informa business

© 2022 selection and editorial matter, **Dave Roberts and Laura Green**, individual chapters, the contributors.

The right of **Dave Roberts and Laura Green** to be identified as the authors of the editorial material, and of the authors for their individual chapters, has been asserted in accordance with sections 77 and 78 of the Copyright, Designs and Patents Act 1988.

British Library Cataloguing-in-Publication Data
A catalogue record for this book is available from the British Library

Library of Congress Cataloging-in-Publication Data
A catalog record has been requested for this book

ISBN: 978-0-8153-6203-6 (hbk)
ISBN: 978-0-8153-6205-0 (pbk)
ISBN: 978-1-351-11347-2 (ebk)

DOI: 10.4324/9781351113472

Typeset in Sabon
by Deanta Global Publishing Services, Chennai, India

Dave: I would like to dedicate this book to my brother Phil and my late sister Jen. The older I get the more I see how important those early years were when we were growing up together

Laura: I'd like to dedicate this book to my partner Andy and my three daughters Martha, Eve and Thea. In addition, to the student nurses who will nurse us all in future years

Contents

List of figures   ix
List of tables   x
List of boxes   xi
List of contributors   xii
Foreword   xiv
Acknowledgements   xvi

1 What is collaborative practice and why is it important in
   palliative care?   1
   Dave Roberts

2 The importance of place: Collaboration across institutional
   boundaries   12
   Laura Green

3 Seeing a familiar face: Collaboration across professional boundaries   26
   Laura Green and Vanessa Taylor

4 Caring for the person in their world: Collaboration in context   38
   Victoria Ali

5 Systems within systems: Collaboration with the family   49
   Linda McEnhill and Patricia McCrossan

6 Building bridges: Collaboration between organisations   59
   Manjula Patel

 7 Psychological care: Everybody's business?   69
    Dave Roberts

 8 Compassionate communities: Working with
    marginalised populations   82
    Aliki Karapliagkou

 9 Collaboration in palliative care: Global perspectives   98
    Dave Roberts, Zipporah Ali, and Brigid Sirengo

10 The future: Developing collaborative palliative care   110
    Dave Roberts

Index   121

Figures

2.1 Professionals who may be involved in Rapid Discharge Planning   21
3.1 The "SWAN" model (courtesy of www.pat.nhs.uk)   35

Tables

3.1 Multiprofessional team involvement   29
6.1 Principles of effective interdisciplinary teamwork   66
9.1 Global surveys of palliative care   100

Boxes

1.1   Effective teamwork requirements   3
1.2   Integrated palliative care: Key domains of care delivery   6
10.1 Core interdisciplinary competencies in palliative care   114
10.2 PACE: 6 steps to success   115
10.3 Palliative care pandemic plan   116

Contributors

Victoria Ali is a Senior Lecturer in Adult Nursing at the University of Huddersfield. Her clinical experience is in oncology and palliative care with a research interest in ethical decision-making at end of life.

Dr Zipporah Ali is the former Executive Director, now advisor to the board, of Kenya Hospices and Palliative Care Association (KEHPCA). She is a board member of several organisations including Alzheimer/Dementia Kenya, Kenya Network of Cancer Organizations, City Cancer Challenge, International Children's Palliative Care Network and the Public Health Palliative Care International. She is a strong advocate for access to quality palliative care in her country and beyond.

Dr Aliki Karapliagkou is Lecturer in Sociology at the University of Bradford. Her research interests include identity transitions at the end of life, bereavement and public health end of life care, and the sociology of health and illness. She focuses her studies upon the lived experiences of marginal and ethnic minority populations, and for that purpose she utilises cultural studies, poststructuralist, and postcolonial literatures.

Patricia McCrossan is a social worker with 18 years of experience in specialist palliative care. She is currently working as Social Work Manager at the North London Hospice and Advanced Practitioner with a hospital discharge team in Hertfordshire. She enjoys teaching with particular interests in narrative, solution focused, systemic and strengths-based models, and loss and bereavement.

Linda McEnhill is CEO of Ardgowan Hospice in Greenock, Scotland. She is the founder of the Network for Palliative Care of People with Learning Disabilities, a trustee of

Hope for Home, a national charity which seeks to enable people with dementia to die in their own "homes" and is also a trustee of Inverclyde CVS.

Manjula Patel is the Chief Executive Officer of Murray Hall Community Trust and has a wealth of experience of working in the voluntary sector including an international charity and local charities. Her doctoral research study with Warwick University is on the development of compassionate communities as a public health approach to end of life care.

Dr Brigid Sirengo, a nurse, midwife, and health visitor with MSc in Palliative Care, was the first Chief Executive of Nairobi Hospice. She had a leading role in the Kenya Hospices and Palliative Care Association. She initiated links with Oxford Brookes University resulting in the Diploma of Higher Education in Palliative Care.

Dr Vanessa Taylor held clinical roles in cancer and palliative care, before moving into higher education with a commitment to educate health professionals about cancer, and palliative and end of life care. Vanessa's published work focuses on: cancer, palliative and end of life care; and evaluation of education and its impact.

Foreword

Leonard Cohen's words "Dance me through the panic till I'm gathered safely in" describe what support really means towards the end of life – collaboratively helping people to dance through the panic. The anxiety that comes with facing mortality.

Collaboration means "work with" from the Latin. "Work with" is so much more than networking, more than understanding. It's joining together to achieve the same goal, sharing a purpose, agreeing a common language whether it's the comfort of a patient in their last hours, calming a conflict within a family, or supporting grief within the wider community.

The UK is blessed with so many services – NHS, charitable, community – but the fragmentation and dissonance of values, targets, and language means that we don't get the best out of these services. The fragmentation of services matches the fragmentation of the body that we have seen in modern medicine. Expert teams focus on body parts but no one looks at the whole patient. Expert teams focus on the patient, but no-one focuses on the whole system – the patient, their family, their social network, their life context.

We need to join these universes – the often hidden social universe and the powerful dominant professional universe. The power has to shift to achieve this collaboration – but in so doing, the energy and the resilience of the whole system could increase!

But true collaboration requires trust, humility, courage, and transparency. Trust that your collaborators will be on the same page as you, humility in that you can't do it all yourself, transparency in sharing what you know, and the courage to let go and recognise your interdependence.

So the chapters in this book give me hope. There are extraordinary examples of new ways of working, of new solutions to ancient problems. We have seen radical collaboration during this terrible pandemic, reduction of bloated bureaucracy, and the melting of barriers. Why fill in a form when you can pick up the phone? There are so many ideas in these chapters that could be scaled up and amplified.

We need to free up healthcare workers to do what they are best at, and open our eyes to new and braver collaborations – moving from person-centred care to network-centred care, embracing new partners, collaborating across professional and global borders, asking not just "what matters", but "who matters" and how can they help?

Dr Ros Taylor MBE DL
Medical Director Harlington Hospice and
Michael Sobell Hospice, Watford
January 2021

Acknowledgements

We would like to thank our colleagues at the Centre for the Advancement of Interprofessional Education (CAIPE), who commissioned this book as part of their series on collaborative practice. Specifically, we thank Marion Helme, Hugh Barr, and Maggie Hutchings for their encouragement, support, and feedback at critical points in the process of writing, editing, and producing this book. We also wish to thank our co-authors for their tenacity, creativity, and collaboration.

Dave would like to thank Mark Foulkes for his advice and feedback on several of the chapters. He thanks his wife Farzaneh for her support during the process of writing and editing. He would also like to thank the many colleagues, students, and patients who have helped to deepen his understanding of palliative care over the years. He has particularly appreciated the many insights he has gained through working with colleagues and students in Africa, and he thanks Brigid Sirengo and Zipporah Ali, contributors to this book, and also Catherine Ajuoga, Jescah Ng'ang'a, Esther Wekesa, John Wekesa, Charles Amoah, Yaw Adu-Gyamfi, and Dela Dzaka, and the late Sobbie Mulindi.

Laura would like to acknowledge her clinical and academic colleagues at the Universities of Manchester and Bradford, and the Continuing Bonds research project team – Dr Karina Croucher, Dr Christina Faull, Dr Jenny Dayes, Dr Lindsey Buster, and Justine Raynsford – for catalysing new ways to think about palliative care, bereavement, and transdisciplinarity. She also thanks her students from the UK and across the world for continually illuminating perspectives, debates, and discussions.

CHAPTER 1

What is collaborative practice and why is it important in palliative care?

....

Dave Roberts

OUTLINE

Palliative care is an essentially collaborative activity. Since the earliest development of the hospice movement, care was organised within teams, making the most of each professional contribution to deliver holistic care of the patient. Dame Cecily Saunders, the founder of contemporary palliative care, was herself an outstanding example of interprofessionalism, training first as a nurse, then medical almoner (equivalent to social worker), before finally training as a doctor, the professional base which gave her the opportunity to develop care for the dying according to her vision. As palliative care has evolved, it has continued to function as a collaboration between different professions, and as a collaboration between patient, family, and professional.

BACKGROUND

As palliative care has moved outside of the hospice base, it has involved collaborations within hospitals, care homes, and primary care, working across professional boundaries and across organisations. This boundary crossing has been characterised as between specialist palliative care staff and generalist care staff, and using a palliative care approach. The following are common definitions of these levels of palliative care work:

- **Specialist palliative care** is provided by specially trained professionals whose primary area of practice is palliative care, whether this is in a hospice, hospital, or community setting. Palliative care specialists also support and educate generalists and those using the palliative care approach.
- **General palliative care** is provided by health and social care staff whose work regularly involves aspects of palliative care, and who have good basic palliative

DOI: 10.4324/9781351113472-1

care skills and knowledge, but this is not their primary responsibility (for example cancer specialist doctors and nurses).

- **Palliative care approach** is the application of palliative care aims, methods and procedures in general (non-palliative care) settings, including acute (hospital), primary care (home), and long term care (nursing and residential care homes).

Collaborative practice is essentially professionals working together towards a common purpose, for the benefit of their patients or clients. When teams work together, their efforts as a team are greater than their individual contributions. Increasingly, we also see collaboration as involving the patient and their family. In the palliative care setting, non-professional volunteers are often part of the team. Collaboration has the meaning of an active and ongoing process, involving people from different backgrounds, working together to solve problems and provide services (Reeves et al., 2010).

Palliative care is well defined, and the following definition from the European Association for Palliative Care (EAPC) emphasises its collaborative nature:

> Palliative care is the active, total care of patients whose disease is not responsive to curative treatment. Palliative care takes a holistic approach, addressing physical, psychosocial and spiritual care, including the treatment of pain and other symptoms. Palliative care is interdisciplinary in its approach and encompasses the care of the patient and their family and should be available in any location including hospital, hospice and community. Palliative care affirms life and regards dying as a normal process; it neither hastens nor postpones death and sets out to preserve the best possible quality of life until death.
>
> *(Radbruch et al., 2010, p. 280)*

The terms palliative care and end of life care are often used interchangeably. However, end of life care refers to the period of months or years when it is apparent that the patient has a life-limiting illness, or more specifically to the care of dying patients in the last hours or days of life. Recently, the inclusive term *Palliative, End of Life and Bereavement care* (PEoLB) has also come into use. Within this book, *palliative care* is used to describe the whole range of palliative care services, unless the discussion is specific to end of life care or bereavement support.

INTERPROFESSIONAL PRACTICE

Collaboration in contemporary palliative care can be viewed within the context of interprofessional practice (IPP). Alternative terminology includes interdisciplinary or multidisciplinary, and the latter term is often used in referring to the multidisciplinary team, or MDT. Strictly speaking, multidisciplinary refers to academic disciplines, though in this context it refers to professional specialisations. Multidisciplinary meetings are one of the key ways in which interprofessional teams operate. Whereas interprofessional working is the norm in specialist palliative care, it may not be in other settings where a palliative care approach is used. It is important to be aware of the different ways in which professionals can work together.

There is a range of terminology that can be used to describe different degrees of working together and integration of professional activity:

- *Teamwork* implies a very close working relationship with a shared sense of team identity.
- *Coordination* is a looser working relationship.
- *Integrated*, as in integrated care pathway, describes activities coordinated along a specific illness trajectory.
- *Networking* is sporadic communication and coordination between groups, when needed.
- *Partnership* may describe the working relationships between two groups.

Alongside these differences, collaboration has value as an overall term for groups working together for a common purpose. The working relationship may be close or looser depending on the nature of the work and the demands that it makes. As a general rule, the more urgent and unpredictable the demands of the work, the greater the need for close teamwork, and where the demands are more routine and predictable, the more suitable a coordinated or networking relationship becomes.

Factors that underlie collaborative practice include communication and decision making, responsibility, accountability, cooperation, assertiveness, autonomy, mutual trust, and respect (Bridges et al., 2011). Teamwork is effective when there are common goals and a sense of shared identity (see Box 1.1).

BOX 1.1 EFFECTIVE TEAMWORK REQUIREMENTS

For professionals to function effectively as a team they need to have:

- Clear goals (focused on patient/client care).
- Shared team identity.
- Shared commitment.
- Clear team roles and responsibilities.
- Interdependence between team members.
- Integration between work practices.

(Reeves et al., 2010)

WHY COLLABORATE?

Traditionally, health care and treatment has been organised according to an acute care model, where discrete conditions were expected to respond to specific interventions leading to a satisfactory outcome. This was associated with a hierarchical structure, often dominated by the medical profession. With the shift to long term conditions, and increasingly complex health and social care management, more diverse teams have become more common, and the emphasis is more on models of collaboration. This offers better opportunities for managing quality and safety, and for better integration of the patient and family into the processes of decision making (Reeves et al., 2010).

There is also evidence that collaborative practices lead to improvements in access to services, better use of specialist services, and a reduction in hospital admissions, length of stay, clinical errors, patient complications, and mortality (WHO 2010). Organisationally, collaboration makes sense as the best way to manage limited resources and maximise the potential input of each member of the interprofessional team.

One of the problems with IPP is that professionals are trained and socialised within their own professional groups, learning the norms and values, alongside professional codes of practice, rules, and regulations. There is therefore the potential for conflict between roles if their professional values or interests are seen to be compromised. This is a particular risk if communication is poor or if roles are not clearly defined, and it can also be exacerbated at times of stress or high demand (Hall 2005).

In addition, professionals may not be taught the range of skills needed to manage complex interprofessional situations. In response to this problem, a number of initiatives have arisen to enable students of different professional groups to learn together: interprofessional education (IPE). This does not replace professional education programmes but enhances them and mirrors the reality of health care practice. It provides opportunities for learning about and with each other, sharing skills and knowledge, and learning to respect each other's roles and values (Bridges et al., 2011). IPE can continue after professional registration, and can include students, professionals, and academics learning together (WHO 2013). There is an overlap between IPP and IPE, in that the practice of working together provides opportunities to learn, so that IPE can function alongside practice (Reeves et al., 2011).

COLLABORATIVE PRACTICE IN PALLIATIVE CARE

Palliative care, with its emphasis on holistic care, is well suited to a collaborative approach. Indeed, the integration of different professionals in the care of the patient and family is both desirable and inevitable. In the words of Radbruch et al.,

> Palliative care is supposed to be provided within a multiprofessional and interdisciplinary framework. Although the palliative care approach can be put into practice by a single person from a distinct profession or discipline, the complexity of specialist palliative care can only be met by continuous communication and collaboration between the different professions and disciplines in order to provide physical, psychological, social and spiritual support.
>
> *(Radbruch et al., 2010, p. 284)*

As palliative care has grown beyond the hospice, and diversified from its earlier focus on cancer, new working relationships have developed, and the distinction between the specialist palliative care practitioner and their generalist colleagues has emerged. These have primarily involved hospital-based colleagues, for example, on oncology wards, and colleagues in primary care. Working across professional boundaries and across different settings is helped by having a sense of common purpose and keeping the interests of the patient and their family at the heart of decision making and care planning.

Effective collaboration is supported by good, clear definition of roles and responsibilities, making the most of opportunities for shared learning and education, good access to specialist palliative care services, and coordinated care (Gardiner et al., 2012). Factors that hinder effective working include the uncertainty of the illness trajectory, often a challenge in non-cancer conditions where the transition to palliative care is less predictable, lack of definition of professional roles, and lack of coordination between professionals (Oishi & Murtagh 2014).

The setting of palliative care delivery also has an impact on collaborative working. Hospital settings, usually involving acute episodes of care, support close working relationships, good communication, and opportunities for learning from each other. However, the busy working environment, with frequent demands and interruptions, can also disrupt communication, leading to misunderstandings or role confusion (Firn et al., 2016).

Within community settings, communication may be more fragmented with less face-to-face interactions. There may be a greater need to schedule meetings, clarify roles, and make opportunities for education and skill-building. The palliative care specialist can work with the generalist by supporting those who are less confident and encouraging more skilled and experienced staff to make the most of their expertise (Firn et al., 2016).

INTEGRATED PALLIATIVE CARE

Palliative care has clear defining features that make it a fundamentally collaborative endeavour. It is person-centred and holistic, family-focused, team-based, and aims for integration with other health services. As such, it can also make a claim for taking an integrative approach, one that has developed in the care of long term conditions. This goes beyond professional teamwork and social inclusiveness to adopt an overall integrated organisation of services for the benefit of patient care. This has become an attractive model as palliative care has increasingly moved outside of its earlier boundaries, to lead care at the end of life in a range of different settings and with diverse groups of professional and lay workers. Hasselaar and Payne (2016) define integrated palliative care:

> Integrated palliative care involves bringing together administrative, organizational, clinical, and service aspects in order to realize continuity of care between all actors involved in the care network of patients receiving palliative

care. It aims to achieve quality of life and a well-supported dying process for the patient and the family in collaboration with all the care givers (paid and unpaid).

(Hasselaar & Payne 2016, p. 8)

den Herder-van der Eerden et al. (2018) suggest that the key to promoting effective integrated care is good organisation of key domains of the care delivery process (see Box 1.2).

BOX 1.2 INTEGRATED PALLIATIVE CARE: KEY DOMAINS OF CARE DELIVERY

(1) Content of care: ensuring that patients receive the right care.
(2) Patient flow: ensuring that the right patients receive care at the right time from the right healthcare professional.
(3) Information logistics: ensuring that the right information is available at the right time.
(4) Availability of resources: ensuring that the right professional and the right medication and equipment are available at the right time.

(den Herder-van der Eerden et al., 2018)

Within the context of palliative services, content of care refers to ensuring those in need of palliative care expertise have access to it, whether by specialist or generalists. Patient flow is concerned with referral systems and how they operate to ensure timely transfer to specialist palliative care services. Information logistics describes a range of communication modes, to ensure decision making is shared and recorded. Resources are a fundamental but problematic issue, particularly when it comes to personnel. This has recruitment and training aspects, in ensuring a competent and well supported palliative care workforce.

In the integrated care model, den Herder-van der Eerden et al. (2018) identified that palliative care is usually carried out by a *core team*, some of whom are specialists, who work closely and within agreed protocols or guidelines. An *extended professional network* includes those who work with the core team as necessary, and may meet occasionally. Whilst they may have some palliative care training, their primary responsibility may not be palliative care; they may for example be a general practitioner, community nurse, or other specialist (e.g. heart failure). However, they know the importance of palliative care, share common values, and have developed trusting relationships with the core palliative care team. The *wider professional community* will also become involved at times with the care of patients. They may, for example, include hospital specialists whose primary function is curative, but are involved in some aspects of the patient's care, e.g. surgery or radiotherapy. The boundaries of these three different groups are permeable: they may join or leave at different points depending on the needs of the patient.

Points of transition, referrals, and discharges, can be a problem as the patient moves across these organisational and professional boundaries. Patients can find these particularly difficult, for example, moving from curative to palliative management, with changes to treatment aims and changes of familiar personnel. Standardisation of practice, by using care pathways or guidelines, is one way to mitigate against this and ensure consistent standards of care and patient experience. However, this is unlikely to be enough on its own, as the wider professional community needs to learn the value of palliative care, for example, through education programmes, and actively engage with it in order for practice to improve (den Herder-van der Eerden et al., 2018).

END OF LIFE CARE POLICY AND INTEGRATED CARE PATHWAYS

Standardised care pathways have become a feature of palliative care in the UK, though their introduction has been incomplete and controversial. The introduction of the *End of Life Care Strategy* (DoH 2008) made end of life care a major priority for the NHS in England, promoting access to high quality care for all people approaching the end of life, irrespective of their circumstances and place of care, through developing a care pathway approach. One driver for this was the high numbers of people dying in hospital in spite of a general wish among the population to die at home. This first major End of Life Care (EoLC) strategy emphasised the coordination of services across all aspects of health care, and this has had a lasting effect on all subsequent policy initiatives.

Other initiatives that have contributed to the development of end of life care include the *Gold Standards Framework* (GSF), a systematic approach to ensuring that people should be able to live and die well in the place and the manner of their choosing. The GSF aims to improve quality of care experienced by people and coordination across boundaries, enabling more people to live well and die well, and reducing hospitalisation. To achieve this, GSF provides training, tools and resources, measures of progress, support, and coaching.

The *Liverpool Care Pathway for the Dying Patient* (LCP) is an approach to care, including a complex set of interventions, developed to replicate within the hospital setting the standard of care for the dying found in hospices. It was put forward as a model of good practice by successive UK national policy frameworks. However, following a series of alarming stories in the media concerning the LCP, Neuberger et al. (2013) were invited to conduct an independent review of the use and experience of LCP in England. They recommended that the LCP be phased out and be replaced by a more individualised approach, and one that emphasised the importance of communication at all stages of the care trajectory.

In response to Neuberger et al. (2013), another independent review by a coalition of 21 national organisations, the Leadership Alliance for the Care of Dying People (LACDP) (2014) published national guidance, *One Chance to Get it Right*, and introduced five priorities for care of the dying person: Recognise, Communicate, Involve, Support, Plan & Do. The National Palliative and EoLC Partnership (2015) published a national framework, *Ambitions for Palliative and EoLC. A national framework for local action 2015–2020*. The framework consists of six ambitions for care: each person seen as an individual; each person gets fair access to care; maximising comfort and wellbeing; care is coordinated; all staff are prepared to care; and each community is prepared to help.

In 2015 the National Institute for Health and Care Excellence (NICE) published an evidence-based guideline *Care of dying adults in the last days of life*. This assists the health professional in recognising the dying phase, monitoring signs of stability or improvement, communicating decisions, and managing the symptoms of the dying person. NICE (2017) also introduced *Quality Standards* for organisations to measure current EoLC service provision and to identify areas for improvement.

The Royal College of Physicians and Marie Curie (2016) conducted an audit of EoLC in hospitals in England. The audit report concluded there have been improvements in all aspects of EoLC in hospitals but variations in provision of services still exist with some services underperforming. The Lancet Oncology Commission has proposed the use of standardised care pathways and multidisciplinary teams to promote the integration of oncology and palliative care. They identify that changes must be made at a system level to achieve this, to coordinate professional activity and develop education programmes, with the goal of improving patient care. They also acknowledge the need for adequate resources, goal setting, and support for better integration (Kaasa et al., 2018).

The NICE (2019) guidance *End of Life Care for Adults: Service Delivery* emphasises the role of electronic information-sharing systems in enabling information to be accessed, updated, and shared efficiently by the different services and organisations involved. It recommends effective coordination of care across teams and settings, including regular discussions and care reviews, and efficient and compassionate transfers between services, ensuring that care packages and equipment are available to enable patients to die in their place of choice.

THE STRUCTURE OF THIS BOOK

This book is designed to address the issues raised by collaboration in the field of palliative and end of life care. The chapters are organised around different settings and working practices, using as their focus the process of working across professional and non-professional boundaries that characterises collaborative practice.

Case studies are provided in Chapters 2 to 9 to illustrate how collaboration works in practice within different contexts and settings. In Chapters 5 and 8, a single extended case study is used to explore in depth the collaborative approach to working with a family and with a community respectively.

The book starts with a focus on interprofessional collaboration in end of life care in Chapters 2, 3, and 4. Chapter 2 discusses working across institutional boundaries, exploring patient journeys as they navigate complex health systems, with reference to the model of integrated palliative care. The chapter also discusses competing ideologies of care that complicate transitions between settings, and highlights examples of good practice in overcoming these challenges.

Chapter 3 addresses working across professional boundaries, highlighting the impact of different professional values. Effective collaboration enhances continuity of care and makes the most of each professional's contribution to meeting common goals. This chapter discusses the challenges of interprofessional working and successful projects.

Chapter 4 is an exploration of the impact of context on interprofessional working. With a focus on the home as the setting for end of life care, it discusses the diversity of what constitutes home for different people, including residential and nursing homes, prisons, and mental health units. It also addresses inequality in access to healthcare, highlighting marginalised groups, and argues for avoiding prior assumptions about people and their needs, and using inclusive language.

Collaboration in palliative care is not only about professionals. Families are an essential part of collaborative working in palliative care, and Chapter 5 focuses on the family as a unit of care and as a system within the health and social care system. It uses a systems approach for analysing family dynamics and working in partnership with families. This chapter argues that the systems approach enables the promotion of family resilience.

Chapter 6 is an analysis of one project that moved outside of traditional professional boundaries and working practices to provide palliative care within a community with a high deprivation index. A novel partnership between a NHS specialist palliative care service and a third-sector organisation delivered two palliative care services. The chapter outlines the features of the partnership that supported an integrated approach, and discusses factors that promote and hinder collaboration.

All team members in palliative care provide some form of psychological care, and Chapter 7 discusses how this can be managed to avoid role conflict and ambiguity. It does this by exploring the use of the NICE four level model of psychological support, distinguishing between different contributions to psychological assessment and intervention. It also addresses the demands of this aspect of palliative care, and the supportive strategies needed to manage this.

Engagement between marginalised communities and palliative care services requires not just knowledge about cultural practices but also understanding of their historical, political, and socio-economic background. Chapter 8 explores, through the findings of one research project, how communities manage end of life within their own resources, based on their unique social circumstances and historical experiences. The public health approach to palliative care and the *Compassionate Cities* and *Communities* movement provide opportunities for palliative care services to understand and develop meaningful partnerships with communities.

Palliative care is a global phenomenon, with great potential for international collaboration. Chapter 9 discusses specific cases and the issues raised by global palliative care. In spite of substantial resource issues, international partnerships and local initiatives have contributed to the rapid development of services in many low- to middle-income countries. This needs to be underpinned by models of sustainable development.

Finally, Chapter 10 looks to the future of collaborative practice in palliative and end of life care. New challenges have arisen as a result of global pandemics, and palliative care continues to adapt to changing circumstances. This will mean working not only across professional boundaries but with family groups and communities, recognising that the home and the local community is the natural place for death, dying, and bereavement.

KEY POINTS

- Collaborative practice in palliative care is well established and continues to develop in new directions in response to the health care environment.
- It can be viewed as a form of interprofessional practice, with which it shares many key characteristics.
- Collaborative practice works well when care is patient- and family-centred, and communication is open and effective.
- Activity should be well organised and coordinated, with clarity of purpose, shared values, and well defined roles and responsibilities.
- Services should be integrated as far as possible for maximum efficiency, though integrated care pathways are still being debated and developed.
- Education is an essential feature of palliative care practice, and opportunities for interprofessional learning should always be sought.
- It is important to remember that different levels of interprofessional involvement, e.g. teamwork or networking, will suit different contexts and situations, and mutual respect is central to collaboration.

REFERENCES

Aldridge, MD, Hasselaar, J, Garralda, E, van der Eerden, M, Stevenson, D, McKendrick, K, Centeno, C, Meier, DE (2016) Education, implementation, and policy barriers to greater integration of palliative care: a literature review. *Palliative Medicine*, 30(3), 224–239.

Bridges, DR, Davidson, RA, Odegard, PS, Maki, IV, Tomkowiak, J (2011) Interprofessional collaboration: three best practice models of interprofessional education. *Medical Education Online*, 16, 1. doi: 10.3402/meo.v16i0.6035

den Herder-van der Eerden, M, van Wijngaarden, J, Payne, S, Preston, N, Linge-Dahl, L, Radbruch, L, Hasselaar, J (2018) Integrated palliative care is about professional networking rather than standardisation of care: a qualitative study with healthcare professionals in 19 integrated palliative care initiatives in five European countries. *Palliative Medicine*, 32(6), 1091–1102. doi: 10.1177/0269216318758194

Department of Health (2008) *End of life care strategy: promoting high quality care for all adults at the end of life*. Department of Health, England.

Firn, J, Preston, N, Walshe, C (2016) What are the views of hospital-based generalist palliative care professionals on what facilitates or hinders collaboration with in-patient specialist palliative care teams? A systematically constructed narrative synthesis. *Palliative Medicine*, 30, 240–256.

Gardiner, C, Gott, M, Ingleton, C (2012) Factors supporting good partnership working between generalist and specialist palliative care services: a systematic review. *British Journal of General Practice*, 62(598), e353–e362.

Hall, P (2005) Interprofessional teamwork: professional cultures as barriers. *Journal of Interprofessional Care*, 19(sup1), 188–196. doi: 10.1080/13561820500081745

Hasselaar, J, Payne, S (2016) *Integrated palliative care*. Radboud University Medical Center, Nijmegen. http://www.insup-c.eu.

Kaasa, S, Loge, JH, Aapro, M, Albreht, T, Anderson, R, Bruera, E, Lundeby, T (2018) Integration of oncology and palliative care: a Lancet Oncology Commission. *The Lancet Oncology*, 19(11), e588–e653. doi: 10.1016/S1470-2045(18)30415-7

National Palliative and End of Life Care Partnership (2015) *Ambitions for palliative and end of life care: a national framework for local action 2015-20*. National Palliative and End of Life Care Partnership. http://www.endoflifecareambitions.org.uk

Neuberger, J, Guthrie, C, Aaronvitch, D, Hameed, K, Bonser, T, Harries, R, Charlesworth-Smith, D, Jackson, E, Cox, D, Waller, S (2013) *More care less pathway: a review of the Liverpool Care Pathway*. Independent Review of the Liverpool Care Pathway.

NICE (National Institute for Health and Care Excellence) (2015) *Care of dying adults in the last days of life*. NICE guideline [NG31]. https://www.nice.org.uk/guidance/ng31

NICE (National Institute for Health and Care Excellence) (2017) *Care of dying adults in the last days of life*. Quality standard [QS144]. https://www.nice.org.uk/guidance/qs144

NICE (National Institute for Health and Care Excellence) (2019) *End of life care for adults: service delivery*. NICE guideline [NG142]. http://www.nice.org.uk/guidance/ng142

Oishi, A, Murtagh, FE (2014) The challenges of uncertainty and interprofessional collaboration in palliative care for non-cancer patients in the community: a systematic review of views from patients, carers and health-care professionals. *Palliative Medicine*, 28(9), 1081–1098.

Radbruch, L, Payne, S, Bercovitch, M, Caraceni, A, De Vlieger, T, Firth, P, Hegedus, K, Nabal, M, Rhebergen, A, Schmidlin, E, Sjøgren, P, Tishelman, C, Wood, C, De Conno, F (2010) White paper on standards and norms for hospice and palliative care in Europe: part 1. *European Journal of Palliative Care*, 17, 22–23.

Reeves, S, Goldman, J, Gilbert, J, Tepper, J, Silver, I, Suter, E, Zwarenstein, M (2011) A scoping review to improve conceptual clarity of interprofessional interventions. *Journal of Interprofessional Care*, 25(3), 167–174.

Reeves, S, Lewin, S, Espin, S, Zwarenstein, M (2010) *Interprofessional teamwork for health and social care*. Blackwell-Wiley, London.

Royal College of Physicians, Marie Curie (2016) *End of life care audit: dying in hospital*. Royal College of Physicians, London.

World Health Organization (2010) *Framework for action on interprofessional education and collaborative practice*. World Health Organization. http://www.who.int/hrh/resources/frame work_action/en/index.html

World Health Organization (2013) *Interprofessional collaborative practice in primary health care: nursing and midwifery perspectives*. World Health Organization. https://apps.who.int/iris/handle/10665/120098

CHAPTER 2

The importance of place

Collaboration across institutional boundaries

....

Laura Green

OUTLINE

Most transitions in a place of care occur during the last three months of life (Abarshi et al., 2010). The majority of these are hospital admissions from a "usual" place of care. This can give rise to problems, potentially jeopardising continuity of care and causing distress to patients and their loved ones. Collaboration between service providers is essential if such transitions are to take place smoothly and provide care that is aligned with patient preferences, clinically appropriate, and effective. This chapter considers the challenges of transitioning between care settings and identifies case studies that illustrate ways in which collaborative practices can be developed in order to achieve integrated and effective care.

BACKGROUND: INTEGRATED PALLIATIVE CARE

Choosing where to die is not easy, yet enabling such choices is central to high quality palliative care. There are multiple factors for patients and their families to consider. What is the likely trajectory of this illness? What is my realistic prognosis? What will happen to me if I become unable to walk, or eat, or speak? Who is available to care for me at home? What are the likely symptoms I will experience? Is there a limit to the clinical interventions that are acceptable to me? What about when I actually die? Who will be there? Can I have as many (or as few) visitors as I like?

During the final months of a person's life, it is likely that in answering some of these questions it will become necessary to transfer from one place to another. A palliative treatment might be indicated for which inpatient admission is required, or the challenges of managing reducing mobility at home might prompt a period of respite in a care home. Or the move could be more permanent; for those people expressing a preference to die in a hospice, for example, moving from home to hospice might be

DOI: 10.4324/9781351113472-2

the last transition made. Every time a person is moved from one setting to another, there is a potential threat to continuity, safety, and wellbeing.

In this chapter we draw on den Herder-Van der Eerden's model of integrated palliative care (2018) to consider care across institutional boundaries:

- Content of care: ensuring that patients receive the right care.
- Patient flow: ensuring that the right patients receive care at the right time from the right healthcare professional.
- Information logistics: ensuring that the right information is available at the right time.
- Availability of resources: ensuring that the right professional and the right medication and equipment are available at the right time.

Content of care

Although most people in the West express a preference to die at home (see for example Munday, Petrova and Dale, 2009; Gomes et al., 2015; Howell et al., 2017) this is not always possible. In the UK, the majority of deaths occur in residential care home settings or in hospitals (ONS, 2015). Hospitals are rarely a preferred place of death, and providing effective end of life care here can be obstructed by the fact that they are in the business of rescuing people (Chapple, 2010). Admission into secondary care requires that a person has a medical problem that can potentially be investigated, diagnosed, and treated in the course of that admission. Hospitals are less well geared up for admissions with multiple, complex problems that might not be amenable to treatment. However, around a third of people in hospital at any one time are likely to be in the last year of life (Clark et al., 2014), so it can be unhelpful to assume that avoiding hospital admission is always possible.

Good communication between community services and acute care means that essential information – be it clinical, related to patient preferences, or to social circumstances that might impact on care – is available to the relevant professionals at the appropriate time. The scenario below in case study 1 illustrates how this can aid (or inhibit) effective palliative care in practice.

Case study 1: Knowing the patient

Dot was discussed at the oncology multidisciplinary team meeting yesterday and it was agreed that her metastatic bowel cancer was not likely to respond to further treatment. She had a diagnosis of dementia, poor renal function, and was unlikely to be strong enough for either systemic chemotherapy or for surgery, which in both cases would have been with palliative intent in any case. Arriving on the Care of the Elderly ward, staff were concerned that she seemed to be in pain. Her eyes were tightly screwed shut and she was moaning continuously, saying "no, no" whilst holding her arms around her middle. The medical and nursing team noted that she was "not for further treatment" and made a decision to commence strong analgesia for her apparent pain. She did not like taking tablets and spat out her oramorph, so the decision was made to commence a continuous subcutaneous infusion (CSCI) with morphine. The following morning, after a settled night, Dot awoke in distress. Confused and thrashing about, staff presumed she was experiencing agitation, and when her CSCI was reprimed they added in some midazolam.

Later that day, she was visited by her Community Matron, Stuart. He had been supporting her and her husband at home for over two years. He was shocked to see the CSCI in place and requested to talk to the medical team. They learned that she had always moaned and closed her eyes when frightened, and that this was not thought to be related to pain. Whenever in an unfamiliar environment, she behaved this way. Stuart explained that she had first been diagnosed with bowel cancer two years ago, and once her bowel habits had been controlled with aperients and she had been on regular paracetamol, she had not experienced any pain according to her family. He strongly believed her current behaviour was to do with being in hospital and urged the discharge team to consider a fast-track discharge. No prognosis had been mentioned. Dot managed to be sent home with the CSCI in place the following day. The following week, Stuart rang the ward to report that Dot was managing without the CSCI, was taking regular paracetamol, and had no signs of distress. She was back at home in her living room, with her husband and family around her.

This scenario is based on actual observations from an ethnographic research project (Green, 2017). It is easy to imagine that without Stuart's intervention, Dot may well have been sedated and given analgesia to the point of unconsciousness, possibly until death. Assumptions were made that her palliative status was equivalent to being in the last days or weeks of life. In fact, Dot lived for a further four months and died at home with input from a community palliative care team and her own district nurses. It is not currently standard practice for community-based healthcare professionals to visit patients from their caseloads whilst in hospital. Stuart visited because he had found out about her admission when he visited her husband, and because he happened to live near the hospital. This serendipitous event meant that the direction of Dot's care was altered.

Issues pertinent to patient care can be overlooked through focusing on immediate needs, coupled with care delivered by a team who may not have access to comprehensive details of the person's clinical and social history. People with life-limiting illness and their families consistently cite that the aspects of care most important are continuity of care, integrated working, and knowing who to contact in case of problems (Middleton-Green et al., 2016; Thomas, Kuhn and Barclay, 2017). Often, hospital admissions are appropriate, necessary, even life-saving, but sometimes they are not. For people with advanced illness, an admission to hospital may actually compound suffering by putting them through investigations or treatments that do not ultimately make any difference to their life expectancy or quality of life. Recognising the transition from curative to palliative care is known to present challenges, particularly where patients have multiple comorbidities. Sometimes no single illness will be expected to cause death, but in conjunction with other comorbidities, people can deteriorate and die relatively unexpectedly.

Patient flow

It is important to be able to identify the point at which hospital is no longer an appropriate place of care in order to expedite discharge or transfer. One of the reasons this may not be achieved is because dying is identified too late. To reduce the occurrence of such instances, collaboration is vital.

Transitioning from curative to palliative treatment can be a difficult time for patients, their loved ones, and for their care providers. There is rarely a clear single point of transition. For example, a person with chronic obstructive pulmonary disease may receive life-saving antibiotics against a backdrop of deteriorating respiratory function. This is a time when decision-making can be contradictory and teams that do not adopt a collaborative approach may find themselves in opposition or conflict. Continuity of care is critical to the patient's experience of transitioning between care settings – but when there are multiple care providers involved, this can become increasingly difficult to achieve.

One of the reasons that planning around place of care can be challenging relates to the difficulty in accurately prognosticating, particularly where a person has a non-malignant condition or is experiencing the general advancing frailty of old age. Prognostication is not an exact science (O'Callaghan et al., 2014), and discharges in the last days of life are to be avoided if at all possible because of the risk of causing or exacerbating distress. Being expected to forge new relationships with a new caregiving team is difficult at the best of times, so being moved when close to death can be traumatic both for patients and for their families.

The strong emphasis on autonomy and choice in end of life care can bring its own challenges. A person may wish to remain at home despite potential risks, and these risks may be physical (such as having a high risk of falling, or unstable symptoms) or psychosocial (such as carer strain or mental health difficulties).

Information logistics

Effective collaboration requires that patient information is available across institutional boundaries. This is particularly important out of hours. If services are unable to access information regarding patients' preferences and current treatment, decisions may be made that are at odds with their wishes or that are clinically inappropriate.

In countries with access to electronic patient records, this is hampered by several factors. Firstly, different services and different regions have historically developed their electronic patient records in a piecemeal way which means that different systems have been implemented, which may or may not be able to communicate with one another.

A second challenge is the issue of data protection. In the UK, the law around data sharing changed in 2018 with the publication of General Data Protection Regulation (GDPR) (Data Protection Act, 2018). The overall goal of this regulation was to ensure that only essential patient information is shared, for specific purposes, and that storage and safety of such data is paramount. There is often a large amount of patient data available, and it is necessary for health professionals to justify disclosure of information and to explain this to patients. Consent must be explicit and not implied. This can be challenging in palliative care settings where patients may have variable mental capacity or be otherwise vulnerable. The notion of the "minimum" necessary amount of information is difficult to interpret in a palliative care context; it may not be clear what information is going to be required now or in the future. The current GDPR arrangement is that patients can opt out of having their information shared, although they may revoke this decision at any time. Clearly if a patient has opted out then this would in reality seriously impair the ability to provide palliative care across institutional boundaries. The change in law is relatively recent, opt-out rates are low, and there is as yet no evidence of this having caused detriment to care. However, concerns have been expressed that a potential rise on opt-out rates may introduce difficulties into care planning and delivery across the spectrum of healthcare (Kuntsman, Miyake and Martin, 2019).

Availability of resources

Although care homes are one of the most common places of death in the UK (Public Health England, 2017) they do not have a good reputation for providing end of life care (Kydd and Wild, 2013). A recent public opinion survey identified that fewer than one in four people would consider moving to a care home. One of the concerns is the lack of specialist palliative care expertise in the staff, particularly in residential homes where there may be no registered nursing staff. Care homes are not as well-equipped to provide holistic palliative care as hospices; hospices can be supported by several hundred volunteers whilst care homes may have fewer than ten (Walshe, 2019). They may also be impacted by more rapid staff turnover (Hospice UK, 2017) meaning that palliative care training and education provided needs to be strategically timed and delivered. The support of specialist palliative care teams is vital; this may take the form of support at a distance – telephone advice and support, signposting or referring to other services – or it may involve more intensive involvement, as in case study 2.

Case study 2: Moving to a care home for end of life care

Bryan was widowed three years ago and has lived alone since then. He has end-stage chronic obstructive pulmonary disease (COPD) and is on long-term oxygen therapy (LTOT). Until last month, he was smoking around 30 cigarettes a day. Over the last few weeks he has become increasingly fatigued. His District Nurses have been visiting to dress a sacral pressure sore. He has become increasingly sleepy, often remaining in bed all day.

One day he expresses to them how much he hates being alone; he misses his wife terribly, and has few other visitors. He cannot manage to prepare even simple meals and drinks for himself. He recognises that there will be a time when even with nursing and healthcare assistants visiting, it will be difficult to stay at home. His District Nurses speak to the hospice admission nurse, and they agree that at present he does not satisfy the admission criteria for a hospice. However, Bryan feels that he cannot stay at home. His local care home is just around the corner. He agrees to be admitted for a period of respite and to see if he might wish to stay there. He does not have current nursing needs so is allocated to a residential care bed, which means that the staff providing care are not qualified nurses.

There are numerous issues within the care home around staff retention, and as a result there are some staff with extensive knowledge of generalist end of life care whilst others have very little knowledge and in fact are worried about how to look after people at the end of life. Over time, and with support from the District Nurses and the GP, Bryan is able to develop an advance care plan that includes his wishes around hospital admission and cardiopulmonary resuscitation. The District Nurses carry out their ongoing input whilst simultaneously supporting and educating the care home staff, so that when the time comes they will be prepared, and will know what they can do, and when and how to contact other services that might be needed, such as hospice at home.

In this case, collaboration requires the development and maintenance of positive relationships with primary care palliative care providers, namely the district nursing teams and – sometimes – specialist palliative care teams. There is no reason why with the involvement of community nurses, a person cannot be well supported and cared for in the last months of life. A recent report on the future of hospice care identified the potential opportunities in the relationships between hospices and care homes (Hospice UK, 2017).

IDEOLOGIES AND INSTITUTIONS

An ideology is a system of "ideas and ideals", it is a "set of beliefs characteristic of a social group or individual" (Oxford University Dictionary Online, 2020). Marx (in

Arthur (ed.), 2004) suggested that the dominant ideology in a society is aligned with the belief system of the most dominant class in that society. Ideologies both shape how we view the world, and how we operate in that world. Different types of care institution adhere to different philosophies of care. Hospitals, for example, have been described as upholding an "ideology of rescue" by Chapple (2010). Her anthropological observations of hospitals suggested that in these settings, death was seen as a "management problem". The "uncharted, untidy and unpredictable" trajectory of dying people posed a challenge to the "finely choreographed" project of rescue.

This ideology continues to exert strong influence in the acute (secondary) care model, particularly in a time of clinical governance and risk management. It can lead to the late identification of dying because of an over-emphasis on medical interventions and investigations, which may no longer be appropriate once the person is approaching the end of life. One palliative care physician once described his role as "rescuing people from the rescuers" (Green, 2017).

In contrast, the ideological routes of older peoples' care lie in the founding mother of geriatric medicine, Marjory Warren. When she adopted responsibility for the management of a workhouse in 1935, Warren found many residents living in squalor, in varying states of neglect and decrepitude. Her development of assessment and management later gave rise to the specialty of geriatric medicine, in which it is essential to recognise and distinguish between reversible and irreversible conditions in order to maximise quality of life. Rehabilitation is central to this approach, where the goal of care is obtaining a balance between appropriate investigations and interventions, and permitting nature to take its course (Barton and Mulley, 2003).

Finally, the ideology of palliative care sees as its focus the avoidance of potentially burdensome interventions and the maximising of quality of life. This emphasises the social, psychological and spiritual aspects of care rather than solely on the physical.

Professionals may adhere closely to one or another of these ideologies, and this may inform their perceptions of the ultimate goal of care for a particular patient. In 2015, the National Palliative and End of Life Care Partnership set out their collective vision and ambitions for end of life care and invited organisations/services to learn how to work together, collectively and differently to achieve these ambitions, finding new ways of delivering better end of life care. To achieve this, it is vital that multiprofessional collaboration and teamworking takes into account the views of each professional in terms of what a "good" outcome might be for a patient. Where a patient has an unpredictable illness trajectory this can prove particularly challenging, so ongoing liaison in the form of multiprofessional team meetings and shared communication and documentation are needed. Ethically sensitive issues such as the withdrawal of treatment, or risk management, can be particularly challenging unless there is overall agreement about whether a patient can be "rescued", or rehabilitated, or whether they are dying.

The following patient journey, case study 3, taken from Green (2017, p. 64) illustrates one example of this, highlighting a transition for Dr Basu whereby he adjusts and realigns his approach in response to this patient's daughter, as it becomes clearer that her father is approaching the end of life.

Case study 3: A patient journey

Dr Basu: "Your dad, he was admitted with a water infection – his blood tests are showing that he is much better and he has had some but not all of his medicine, because he pulls the cannula out. The only thing he's had since admission is fluid. I know he is 94 but if we don't give him food soon his body will break down, his albumin is already very low and this will get worse. Speech and Language Therapy Team (SALT) saw him and think that if he eats food it will go into his lungs and cause a chemical pneumonia which is not nice, so there is a big question mark about how now we are going to feed him. If it is by mouth it is a big risk, a big danger. The other better option from a nutritional position would be an NG tube. This is not easy because we have to insert it blind – we would withdraw some gastric fluid and test it to make sure that it is in the right place, and he would have an X-ray to be certain it has passed into his stomach. Antibiotics will be much easier to give this way, but the main problem is that he might pull this out. If he does, we will put it back in again, and if he pulls it out we would put it in again but with a clip to hold it in his nose. A third option is a PEG feed, but this is a very drastic option."

Next, he explains the procedure…"we use a light to locate…there is a string… the catheter is withdrawn…the tube is inserted… The advantage here is that you can maintain nutrition. There are some side effects…infection, pulling it out…usually this is done as a last resort", concluding with: "We thought it would be nice before we take action to talk to you"

Daughter: "But yesterday he had shepherd's pie…it's not very pleasant, the thought of having a tube"

Dr Basu: "But to keep someone alive they can only be kept alive for a few days on fluids. We need to think about quality of life. Is he independent?"

Daughter: "I've noticed since my mum's died that he's sort of given up"

Dr Basu: "Has he ever expressed that he's had enough?"

Daughter: "Yes, he has"

Dr Basu: "We try and prolong life with any means we have as doctors. We could take a risk, perhaps give him food and see. If he gets pneumonia he has had a good life but now as you say he is lonely…on the other hand though, he is improving. Confusion is much better and whether he has underlying dementia is another question."

Daughter: "I don't know how he would react"

Dr Basu: "I think of it as a battlefield, when we have someone in front of me who is moribund we do everything. But my other hat is as a human being…he's 94, lives alone, wife died…is it treating with all the tubes and things that are giving more trouble? The only reason I support the feeding is that he wasn't bedbound, he was mobile. If he had been bedbound, incontinent, needing all cares, I would have been different. I will be guided by you. We can take a risk and feed him by mouth"

Daughter: "It's difficult, isn't it? How long would it be for? Forever?"

Dr Basu: "It's not a pleasant thing, he might pull it out so we'd put a bridle in on the third time and by that time we would make a decision about PEG feeding. IF the tube stays properly…by Monday if we still have to feed him by tube, if he pulls it out at least we'll have done something"

Daughter: "It's difficult, isn't it? Could we not give him a try with food?"

Dr Basu: "Yes, I am probably insisting a bit much…yes if that is the feeling we will try food"

In this example, the physician's discomfort is clear. He does not know Ned, or his daughter, and is trying to glean as much information as possible from this consultation with regards to the appropriate way to proceed.

SOLUTIONS AND INNOVATIONS

The need to enhance communication between clinical settings has been addressed by a number of service developments. The following section presents three UK-based initiatives that seek to tackle some of the challenges outlined above: Rapid Discharge Planning (or "Fast Track"), Integrated Hospice Services, and Telemedicine.

Rapid Discharge Planning (RDP) is a model of care recently introduced in the UK in which a dying patient, expressing a wish to die at home, is enabled to experience a rapid and coordinated discharge from hospital to home. Also known as "Fast Track", RDP provides a structure for ensuring that all elements required for a smooth discharge are appropriately coordinated. RDP is perhaps a paradigm example of where collaboration across boundaries is at its most vital. Transitioning towards dying tends to be unpredictable, and when dying is eventually diagnosed there is often a very limited time window for discharging a person to their home. The most important element of RDP is arguably the timely recognition of dying, as this means that valuable time is not lost and allows for coordination of the remaining elements of discharge. A wide variety of professionals within the hospital and community must come together to facilitate RDP. The figure below broadly identifies professionals who may be involved in the Rapid Discharge process and outlines key roles.

This is by no means an exhaustive list; additional specialist or generalist professionals may become involved at different times. It can be a baffling time for patients, families, and staff. RDP algorithms have been developed that facilitate interprofessional understanding of the process (for an example, see NHS Greater Glasgow & Clyde, 2019).

Integrating hospice services. UK hospices predominantly operate in ways that support and supplement other providers. In addition, some also supplant local services, taking over direct responsibility and funding in-patient care. They all contribute to integration with local services, with greater blurring of boundaries than defined by the original model. Integrated care offers the necessary flexibility to respond to changes in patient needs, however, constraints from funding drivers and a lack of clear responsibilities in the UK can result in shortfalls in optimal service delivery. Integrating hospice care with local healthcare services can help to address demographic changes, predominantly more frail older people, and disease factors, including the needs of those with non-malignant conditions. This model, tested in the UK, could serve as an example for other countries.

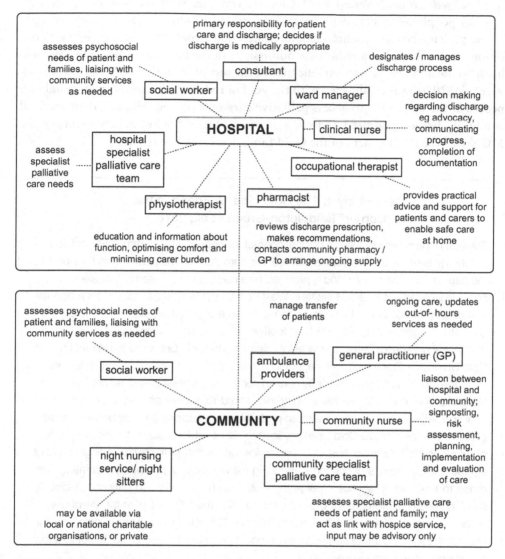

FIGURE 2.1 Professionals who may be involved in Rapid Discharge Planning

Payne et al (2017) propose a stepped model of integration between hospices and local health and care providers. Termed "InSup-C" (Integrated Palliative Care in Cancer and Chronic Conditions), this model describes three levels of engagement, termed "support", "supplant", and "supplement". These layers are best conceptualised as cumulative; supporting existing services means that resources are offered to assist others to provide palliative care. At the next level, supplanting existing services means adding to them according to need; an example might be providing bereavement support for family members or loaning specialist equipment. The third level involves the hospice taking on full clinical responsibility for care, as might be seen when a person is cared for in an in-patient specialist palliative care setting.

Managed Clinical Networks (MCN) are one means of tackling obstacles that arise as people move between clinical settings. In Bradford, UK, an audit of electronic patient records (unpublished) identified that people with non-malignant conditions tended to have more hospital admissions in the last year of life, and were less likely to die at home – a pattern reflective of the rest of the UK. The MCN (Bradford, Airedale, 2020) was established with the goal of reducing this inequity and enabling people at the end of life to access palliative care services regardless of their medical condition, based upon need and not diagnosis. One of the key achievements of the MCN was the development of the Gold Line, described in case study 4.

Case study 4: The Gold Line "A Friend in the Corner" (Middleton-Green et al., 2016)

The Gold Line service is a single point of contact for people in the community identified as potentially being in the last year of life. It offers care coordination, advice and support to the patients and their carers and is provided by a nursing team based at the teleconsultation hub in Airedale General Hospital in West Yorkshire, UK. The service covers a population of around 500,000. These areas comprise an area of urban deprivation and ethnic diversity, villages and towns with low deprivation and high proportions of older people and a rural hinterland. Patients eligible for referral to the Gold Line were those meeting the Gold Standards Framework criteria, not just those eligible for Specialist Palliative Care.

In the region, all GPs, community nursing services, specialist palliative care teams and the Gold Line team use an online electronic record to access and record patient data, enabling sharing of information between professions and across services boundaries with patient consent. Calls to Gold Line may lead to direct advice, referral to another service, or admission to hospital or hospice. The service means that patients had a single point of contact for any queries or concerns, reducing the numbers of potentially frustrating calls made to the "wrong" service. Staff at the Gold Line have access to patients' electronic medical record, so the patient did not need to relay the full story over the telephone. A recent evaluation highlighted that approximately 40% of queries were handled by the nurses; the remainder required arranging a home visit from a nurse or doctor, or in a few occasions, an ambulance was called.

Initial evaluation found that it was not only the access to clinical advice that was valued, but the emotional reassurance of being able to contact someone who could access information about the person and knew their story and their preferences. Some participants found it invaluable when experiencing exacerbations of symptoms such as breathlessness, for advice and support regarding non-pharmacological management of their symptoms. Significantly, use of the service over time enabled patients to build up rapport with the Gold Line team, and even though their care was being provided by a range of providers across a range of settings, this continuity was highly valued. Initial data appeared to show lower rates of unplanned hospital admissions in patients on the Gold Line register, compared with patients who could not access this service.

Telehealth – the exchange of data between a patient and healthcare professionals – is a key priority in current health policy in developed countries such as the UK (Kidd et al., 2010). It also has great potential to enhance care in underserved communities across the globe (WHO, n.d.). Yet its uptake in palliative care services is patchy amid concerns about data security and worries about losing the "personal" aspects of patient-professional relationships. Studies identify that building an evidence base for the effectiveness of telehealth in palliative care has been hampered by challenges in research methods, bias in studies, and differences in the use of patient-reported outcomes as a mode of evaluation (Wootton, 2012; Taylor et al., 2014).

KEY POINTS

- This chapter has addressed some of the challenges in providing collaborative palliative care across institutional boundaries.
- The journey of a person with a life-limiting illness is uncertain, and needs may change in unpredictable ways.
- Collaborative care in such circumstances needs to feel seamless to the patient and their family, who may well be overwhelmed with the sheer number and variety of different professionals and services they encounter.
- "Behind-the-scenes" communication is vital, and central to this is the need for each member of the team to be aware of the role, scope, and capacity of the others.
- The structure of services may preclude the option of formal multiprofessional meetings, so developing effective collaborative practice requires sustainable communication within and between key players in the range of caregiving teams.
- There are a number of potential solutions to existing challenges, and future work must focus upon the need to simplify and streamline the patient journey.

REFERENCES

Abarshi, E, et al. (2010) Transitions between care settings at the end of life in the Netherlands: results from a nationwide study. *Palliative Medicine*, 24(2), 166–174. doi: 10.1177/0269216309351381

Barton, A, Mulley, G (2003) History of the development of geriatric medicine in the UK. *Postgraduate Medical Journal* 79, 229–234.

Bradford, Airedale, Wharfedale and Craven Palliative Care Managed Clinical Network (2020) *Managed clinical network, managed clinical network homepage*. Available at: http://www.palliativecare.bradford.nhs.uk/Pages/Home.aspx.

Chapple, H. (2010) *No place for dying: hospitals and the ideology of rescue*, Left Coast Press, Walnut Creek Illinois

Clark, D, et al. (2014) Imminence of death among hospital inpatients: prevalent cohort study. *Palliative Medicine*, 28(6), 1–6. doi: 10.1177/0269216314526443

Gomes, B, et al. (2015) Is dying in hospital better than home in incurable cancer and what factors influence this? A population-based study. *BMC Medicine*. doi: 10.1186/s12916-015-0466-5

Green, L (2017) *Here there is nobody: an ethnographic of older peoples' end-of-life care in hospital.* University of Bradford: Bradford, UK.

den Herder-van der Eerden, M, et al. (2018) Integrated palliative care is about professional networking rather than standardisation of care: a qualitative study with healthcare professionals in 19 integrated palliative care initiatives in five European countries. *Palliative Medicine,* 1091–1102. doi: 10.1177/0269216318758194

Hospice UK (2017) *Role of specialist palliative care in care homes.* Available at: https://www.hospiceuk.org/about-hospice-care/media-centre/press-releases/details/2017/08/09/new-report-highlights-the-role-of-specialist-palliative-care-support-to-care-homes-in-delivering-high-quality-end-of-life-care.

Howell, DA, et al. (2017) Preferred and actual place of death in haematological malignancy. *BMJ Supportive and Palliative Care,* 7(2). doi: 10.1136/bmjspcare-2014-000793

Kidd, L, et al. (2010) Telehealth in palliative care in the UK: a review of the evidence. *Journal of Telemedicine and Telecare,* 16(7), 394–402. doi: 10.1258/jtt.2010.091108

Kuntsman, A, Miyake, E, Martin, S (2019) Re-thinking digital health: data, appisation and the (im)possibility of "opting out". *Digital Health.* doi: 10.1177/2055207619880671.

Kydd, A, Wild, D (2013) Attitudes towards caring for older people: literature review and methodology. *Nursing Older People,* 25(3), 22–27. Available at: http://www.ncbi.nlm.nih.gov/pubmed/23646417.

Middleton-Green, L, et al. (2016) "A friend in the corner": supporting people at home in the last year of life via telephone and video consultation—an evaluation. *BMJ Supportive & Palliative Care.* p. bmjspcare-2015-001016. doi: 10.1136/bmjspcare-2015-001016.

Munday, D, Petrova, M, Dale, J (2009) Exploring preferences for place of death with terminally ill patients: qualitative study of experiences of general practitioners and community nurses in England. *BMJ (Clinical Research Ed.).* Munday, Daniel, Health Sciences Research Institute, Warwick Medical School, University of Warwick, Coventry, United Kingdom, CV4 7AL: British Medical Association, 339(7714). Available at: http://d.munday@warwick.ac.uk.

NHS Greater Glasgow & Clyde (2019) *Rapid discharge guidance for patients who are in the last days of life.* Available at: https://www.palliativecareggc.org.uk/wp-content/uploads/2013/11/Rapid_Discharge_Algorithm_030317.pdf (accessed 17 September 2020).

O'Callaghan, A, et al. (2014) Can we predict which hospitalised patients are in their last year of life? A prospective cross-sectional study of the Gold Standards Framework Prognostic Indicator Guidance as a screening tool in the acute hospital setting. *Palliative Medicine,* 28(8), 1046–1052. Available at: http://search.ebscohost.com/login.aspx?direct=true&db=rzh&AN=103884325&site=ehost-live.

ONS (2015) *National survey of bereaved people (VOICES), 2014,* available at https://www.ons.gov.uk/peoplepopulationandcommunity/healthandsocialcare/healthcaresystem/bulletins/nationalsurveyofbereavedpeoplevoices/england2015 "Ideology" (2020) In *Oxford Online Dictionary.* Retrieved from https://en.oxforddictionaries.com/definition/ideology

Payne, S, et al. (2017) Enhancing integrated palliative care: what models are appropriate? A cross-case analysis. *BMC Palliative Care.* BioMed Central Ltd., 16(1). doi: 10.1186/s12904-017-0250-8

Public Health England (2017) *The role of care homes in end of life care briefing 2 - place and cause of death for permanent and temporary residents of care homes, briefing.* Available at: https://assets.publishing.service.gov.uk/government/uploads/system/uploads/attachment_data/file/828122/Briefing_2_Place_and_cause_of_death_for_permanent_and_temporary_residents_of_care_homes.pdf (accessed 27 May 2020).

Taylor, J, et al. (2014) Examining the use of telehealth in community nursing: identifying the factors affecting frontline staff acceptance and telehealth adoption. *Journal of Advanced Nursing*, 71(2), 326–337. doi: 10.1111/jan.12480

Thomas, T, Kuhn, I, Barclay, S (2017) Inpatient transfer to a care home for end-of-life care: what are the views and experiences of patients and their relatives? A systematic review and narrative synthesis of the UK literature. *Palliative Medicine*. SAGE Publications Ltd., 31(2), 102–108. doi: 10.1177/0269216316648068.

United Kingdom Government (2018) *Data protection act.*

Walshe, C (2019) Seminar, in Cicely Saunders Institute Open Seminar Series.

WHO (n.d.) *Health and sustainable development: telehealth.*

Wootton, R (2012) Twenty years of telemedicine in chronic disease management–an evidence synthesis. *Journal of Telemedicine and Telecare*, 18(4), 211–220. doi: 10.1258/jtt.2012.120219.

CHAPTER 3

Seeing a familiar face

Collaboration across professional boundaries

....

Laura Green and Vanessa Taylor

OUTLINE

This chapter focuses on the importance of effective multiprofessional teamworking for achieving the benefits of holisitic care for people with palliative and end of life care needs. Drawing on den Herder-Van der Eerden et al.'s (2018) model of integrated palliative care, this chapter relates to "patient flow" defined as ensuring the right patients receive care at the right time from the right healthcare professional. We identify the strengths, tensions, and challenges for collaboration across professional boundaries as service providers seek ways to co-ordinate the delivery of individualised, competent, confident, and compassionate palliative and end of life care. Recognising the tension between different ideologies of care and the need for effective multiprofessional team working is seen as means of reducing fragementation and duplication of care in a system where there are multiple "entry points" for patients. In this chapter, we explore the concepts of boundaries, roles, and teamworking in the delivery of palliative and end of life care. First, we consider definitions of team and teamwork and explore the importance of collaborative palliative care across disciplines and professions. Next, we examine the tensions and challenges. Through case studies, the value of collaboration by professionals is illustrated. New ideas about teams and co-ordination from the perspective of patient and carer involvement are discussed.

BACKGROUND

Delivering person-centred, holistic care through multiprofessional teamwork is a hallmark of palliative and end of life care. Working in teams has been, and continues to be, an integral part of the philosophy of palliative care, enshrined in its standards, and embedded in its practice (Department of Health, 2008; UK National Palliative

DOI: 10.4324/9781351113472-3

and End of Life Care Partnership and National End of Life Care Programme, 2015; National Institute for Clinical Excellence (NICE), 2019; NHS England, 2020). The palliative care "team" comprises different professions and disciplines who draw on their specialist knowledge and skills to meet the range of changing physical, psychological, and social needs of patients and their wider social network (Saunders, 2001). The "team" has, however, changed considerably since the traditional model of palliative care was developed in hospices. Palliative care has evolved and specialist services can now be found in public and charitable funded primary, secondary, and community settings.

Building relationships and working collaboratively with professionals in other services, agencies, and specialities across the health and social care system is needed to ensure each person with a life-limiting condition has fair access to good end of life care (Hall and Payne, 2015).

There has been a shift in policy towards acknowledging inequities in access to palliative and end of life care based on diagnosis. This shift is embodied in the End of life Care (EoLC) programme endorsed by the Department of Health. The EoLC programme aims at providing more choice and improving the quality of end of life care for every person irrespective of diagnosis or place of death. The uncertainty about prognosis for some conditions and openness to discussions about dying and death can, however, challenge teams providing palliative and end of life care, requiring professions within different specialities to engage with, and explore, their professional values, philosophy, and practices alongside those underpinning palliative and end of life care. Professional boundaries of expertise and claims to specialist knowledge and skills may be challenged. Furthermore, the roles and responsibilities of health and social care professionals have evolved with the expectation that all staff are able to provide a level of palliative and end of life care. The defined roles and responsibilities which distinguished the contribution of each member of the palliative care team are also becoming blurred through developments including, for example, advanced clinical practice roles which have expanded levels of autonomy, skills, and decision-making for nursing and allied health professionals. Teamworking in palliative care is, therefore, not straightforward, as the boundaries of place, professional roles, and team membership evolve aiming to deliver person-centred holistic palliative care accessible to all who need it.

TEAMWORKING IN PALLIATIVE CARE

Teams are often defined as a group of people with diverse skills who come together to work towards a common goal or purpose (Katzenbach and Smith, 1993). A team is committed to a common purpose, set of performance goals, and approach for which they hold themselves mutually accountable. Katzenbach and Smith (1993) describe the essence of a team as common commitment. Without it, groups perform as individuals; with it, they become a powerful unit of collective performance. This kind of commitment requires a purpose in which team members can believe. Similarly, Farsides (2006) considers that palliative care teams may be more than professionals with different skills working together for shared goals. Palliative care teams may identify themselves as part of a social movement which shares a common philosophy, driven by values, that are strongly articulated and enacted by its practitioners. The benefits of this approach are increasing the scope of the service offered; management of workload; support of colleagues; and cross-fertilisation of ideas, skills, and knowledge (Øvretveit, 1995). Teamworking can enable high-quality decisions to be made in complex, demanding situations required for person-centred care. These advantages indicate, therefore, the potential for interprofessional teamworking to raise the standard of quality of patient care and family support beyond that which could be provided by individual professionals.

Hall (2006) argues that, in order for interprofessional teams to function collaboratively, members must understand the tenets from which each professional operates. Values are seen as central to a professional culture into which new recruits are socialised through the modelling of ways of thinking and behaving. Established professionals will have a strong professional identity based on their skills, values, and ways of thinking from which they assess and deliver care to patients. Good teamwork, therefore, requires professionals to make explicit their values and ways of thinking and to use their strengths inherent in their professional identity, to effectively share them with the team and patient to meet the common goal of palliative and end of life care according to patient and family needs.

CHALLENGES

Patients with palliative and end of life care needs and their families want to be seen holistically and for health and social care professionals to work with them to manage their physical, emotional, psychological, social, and spiritual needs. They also expect teams and services to work across the health and social care system seamlessly; across the boundaries of primary, secondary, and community services, specialist and generalist services; and NHS and private, independent, and voluntary organisations. System, organisational, and team fragmentation are, therefore, a risk to effective teamworking and, for the patient, risk the opportunity to maximise their comfort and well-being.

The previous chapter considered some of the issues arising from transitions in place of care, including documentation, translation of goals of care, and the importance of continuity. Patients being cared for by multiprofessional teams can find it a challenging experience. Even where there is a common goal of providing optimal patient-centred care, patients can find the experience confusing, disorientating, and difficult to navigate. Table 3.1 illustrates the potential number of different members of the multiprofessional team over a one-week period for a patient participant, "Vincent" (not his real name) in an ethnographic study of older peoples' experiences at the end of life (Green, 2017).

Whilst it is not possible for patients who have complex needs to have these needs met by a single professional, it is vital to ensure that care is provided by a cohesive team familiar to the patient, if the goals of care are to be achieved. One of the issues

TABLE 3.1 Multiprofessional team involvement

Issue	Wishes to go home	Pain	Low mood following bereavement	Poor appetite	Dying phase
Members of staff	Social worker, occupational therapist, physiotherapist, pharmacist, discharge coordinator, care home manager	Doctors, nurses, student nurse, pharmacist	Doctors, nurses, social worker, psychiatry liaison worker, palliative care specialist nurse	Nurses, healthcare support workers, mealtime volunteers, dietician, speech and language therapist	Doctors, nurses, chaplaincy, mortuary, porter, bereavement nurse

identified in the above study was the potential for goals of care to be *implicit*, rather than explicitly stated, documented, and discussed. It is only through effective communication that any misalignment in goals of care can be identified and acted upon. For example, a social worker may work towards a goal of safe and timely discharge, whilst a doctor may be acting upon the most recent set of blood results indicating that a patient's medical condition is not yet stable enough for discharge, or indeed that their deterioration suggests that they may not be able to go home at all.

Potential barriers to person-centred holistic care include limiting working to within one's own professional boundaries. For example, a medical team may be working to stabilise a patient's condition and, because the patient is not considered to be "medically fit" for discharge, the patient will not be referred to a social worker. Once they are medically fit, however, the discharge coordinator needs to identify needs and make further referrals (for example, for any aids and adaptations required at home). This can mean that, by the time the patient is able to go home, a significant delay may have arisen. In some cases, for patients with palliative and end of life care needs, this delay can be the difference between going home and dying in hospital. To address this, it is vital that early communication, collaboration, and referral occurs when the patient first comes into contact with the team and a key contact is identified for the patient and their informal carers.

Across the world, the need for palliative care is increasing, and this includes the increased prevalence of patients with multiple comorbidities. In these cases, there may be a need to involve multiple clinical and care specialities which may be confusing for patients. It is, therefore, crucial to recognise and prevent reductive approaches to care within clinical speciality silos which may lead to missed opportunities or episodes of care, or breakdown in end of life care delivery.

SUPPORTING ONE ANOTHER

As clinical medicine advances and people can be kept well, and alive for longer, it becomes increasingly necessary for different clinical specialisms to be able to work together to ensure optimal care, particularly at the end of life. Geriatricians, cardiologists, palliative care, respiratory physicians, and others all have highly valuable skills and knowledge, but these can only be drawn upon for patient benefit if they are synchronised and collaborative.

Good teamwork requires professionals from different services, specialties, and professional backgrounds to make explicit their values and ways of thinking and to use the strengths inherent in their professional identity, to effectively share them with the team and patient to meet the common goal of palliative and end of life care. Different specialities may, however, have fundamentally different beliefs about care, underpinned by different professional ideologies.

Professional training and ideologies often interpret patient outcomes in different ways. Interprofessional education is one way in which it has been suggested that health and social care professionals can be supported to understand each other's roles in care. One small study of interprofessional palliative care in the home settings identified key concepts that appear to underpin successful collaboration, include sharing of responsibilities and decision-making, partnerships established on mutual trust, interdependency among providers to reach common goals, and shared power among team members (Shaw et al., 2016).

In the community setting, facilitating collaborative approaches has been aided by development and adoption of frameworks such as the Gold Standards Framework (Thomas et al., 2007; Thomas and Lobo, 2011) and the "Six Steps to Success in End of Life Care" (O'Brien et al., 2016). The NICE Guidelines on supportive and palliative care (National Institute for Clinical Excellence (NICE), 2004) recommend that teams must work together to provide continuity for patients and their loved ones. One of their recommendations is the identification of a "key worker" whose role includes the coordination of care and cooperation between all those involved in the disease trajectory. Given the number of professionals, practitioners, carers, and health and social care services contributing to patient care at the end of life, the key worker role can be a familiar face and contact for patients and their families. Although these guidelines are specific to care of people with cancer, the principles are relevant to end of life care regardless of the diagnosis. There is some debate with regards to who is best placed to be a key worker. It is known that most of the last year of life is spent at home, and therefore in many areas the key worker is ideally a general practitioner (GP) or district nurse. However there are times when care may be taken over, for example if a patient deteriorates and a prolonged hospital admission results. Research by Brogaard et al. (2011) identified that disagreement between patients and relatives regarding who the key worker is highlights a need to develop clear outlines about the expectations of this role.

COLLABORATIVE PALLIATIVE CARE IN NON-MALIGNANT CONDITIONS

A narrative synthesis by Oishi & Murtagh (2014) identified that there are particular challenges associated with the provision of multiprofessional care for people with non-malignant conditions, including varying understanding of the role of the general practitioner (GP). Whilst patients appear to value the time and accessibility of GPs in the community, there is also ambivalence about a lack of disease-specific knowledge and whether or not a hospital admission is indicated in exacerbations of existing conditions. Perceptions of the nurses' role were similarly unclear; some patients considered the nurses' role to be task-orientated, whilst others valued the extra time that some nurses were perceived to have to talk about difficult subjects. GPs in these studies considered that nurses were in key positions to act as coordinators and educators for people with non-malignant conditions. Specialist nurses were seen variously as a "hands-off" resource for education and advice regarding medicines, and there was some ambivalence when specialist nurses took on a direct role with patients, with some generalist nurses in the community describing feeling "sidelined" or disempowered. Oishi & Murtagh (2014) identified a number of challenges in developing and improving the provision of collaborative palliative care for people with non-malignant conditions. Specialist doctors were perceived by patients as being difficult to access, whilst GPs reported feeling sidelined by those in the palliative care specialty.

The study highlighted the "reciprocal nature of expectations and concerns between carers, patients and HCPs" (Oishi and Murtagh, 2014, p. 1094). Interestingly, patients and carers did not identify any expectations that primary care nurses fulfilled a role in palliative care, despite having identified concerns about continuity of care. This suggests that patients, and potentially families, are unaware of the potential role played by community nurses in palliative care. There is a need for openness and clarity about role boundaries; too rigid boundaries can disempower and disenfranchise primary care-giving teams, whilst boundaries that are unclear can lead to confusion for patients and professionals alike. A key recommendation for development of these relationships includes raising the profile of the advisory capacity of specialist nurses and doctors. This would capitalise on the accessibility and continuity of relationships with GPs and nurses in primary care, whilst ensuring that the quality of care is maximised.

One of the challenges that seems to particularly impact on people with non-malignant conditions is that of clinical uncertainty (Cousin et al., 2013; Oishi and Murtagh, 2014; Sharp et al., 2018). This can impact on transitions of care, identification of appropriate key workers, and the acceptability of the terminal nature of some conditions by patients and their loved ones. Further research into agile approaches to navigating unpredictable disease trajectories is indicated.

PATIENTS AS PARTNERS: PATIENTS AND
FAMILIES AS MEMBERS OF THE TEAM

The role of patients and families in interprofessional collaboration is frequently unclear and can be highly variable (McDonald and McCallin, 2010). Patients and families may not wish to participate in decision-making, particularly around sensitive issues such as resuscitation. Indeed, some family members report heightened anxiety (Heyland et al., 2009) especially when this discussion appears to come "out of the blue". There is a preference for initiation of such conversations to come from a trusted person rather than a stranger, and for timing of this to be carefully individualised.

TRANSLATION ACROSS BOUNDARIES

Finally, interprofessional collaboration requires that we develop our awareness of how certain issues translate (or not) across professional boundaries. Terms that may be used every day in the professional rhetoric may have fundamentally different meanings to different professionals. The impact of professional socialisation into our understanding of terms and phrases cannot be underestimated, particularly in its potential impact on patients. Consider the oft-cited phrase "there is nothing more that we can do". Whilst this has thankfully become more rarely seen in practice, it has historically been a relatively acceptable way for clinicians to communicate to patients and their families that no further active treatment is possible for their condition – essentially, that they cannot be cured. Although ostensibly true from the perspective of the condition, there is of course always something that we can do. This is where collaboration and teamworking, to deliver palliative and end of life care, enable patients and their families to access the kind of holistic individualised care that is required. Other terms, such as "palliative", "end of life", "end-stage disease", and "terminal" are also commonly misunderstood between and even within professions. Clarity at all points is required, and it is important that team members involved are using similar language when communicating with patients and their lay carers.

LEARNING FROM PRACTICE

To address some of the issues discussed above, innovation in clinical practice is key. The next section outlines two such projects and services, in case studies 1 and 2, to highlight some ways in which interprofessional collaboration can be enhanced.

Case study 1: Heart failure and end of life care – The "Better Together" Project

In two UK NHS Primary Care trusts (Bradford and Poole) the "Better Together" project aimed to address the inequity in accessing palliative care experienced by people with heart failure (Pattenden et al, 2014). This pilot study examined the provision of palliative care to people with advanced congestive cardiac failure. The home-based palliative care services were coordinated by heart failure nurse specialists (HFNSs) using Marie Curie nurses and healthcare assistants, as part of the multiprofessional team.

Measures of success of the "Better Together" project included whether or not the person was able to die in their preferred place of death, and to consider whether collaborative provision of palliative care alongside heart failure specialists was cost-effective. Although cost-effectiveness was not definitively proven, there was a significant increase in the proportion of people who died at home compared to those receiving no palliative care.

The collaboration in Bradford built on existing relationships between heart failure nurse specialists and specialist palliative care services. The heart failure nurses held a regular support group for patients in the Day Therapy Unit of a hospice, with patients being referred as needed for additional support as indicated. The HFNSs were invited to attend the community palliative care team's regular multidisciplinary team meetings (MDTs). HFNSs attended formal educational events organised by the palliative care service and vice versa. Practice-based education for primary care staff was delivered jointly by the HFNSs and a palliative care consultant. This allowed discussion of symptom control issues that the HFNSs did not feel competent to facilitate.

Case study 2: Collaboration in times of disaster – Northern Care Alliance: Swans and Cygnets

The SWAN Model of Care in use across the Northern Care Alliance (2020) seeks to support and guide the care of patients and their loved ones at the end of life and after they have died. With the advent of the COVID-19 pandemic, it soon became apparent that not only would the number of deaths increase greatly, but that the measures necessary for limiting the spread of the pandemic would mean that many people in acute hospitals and within the community would be unable to be with their loved ones at the end of life. Concurrently, a number of health and allied healthcare professionals were informed that the usual roles would not be operational during the pandemic, in order to optimise infection control. This group included speech and language therapists, pre-operative assessment nurses, and research nurses. This group of professionals were invited to join an existing team known as the "SWAN" team.

As illustrated by Figure 3.1, the SWAN team's remit encompassed end of life care and bereavement care. However the advent of COVID-19 and the resultant restrictions on visiting rules within the hospital meant that the service needed to adapt to the new situation to ensure, as far as possible, that the goals and values of the SWAN team could be continued. The new members of the team were called "cygnets" to emphasise their role allied to the SWAN team, and their role was threefold. Firstly, they aimed to support clinical staff across the patch with provision of end of life and bereavement care. Secondly, they were trained to support patients at the end of life to try and ensure that nobody died alone. Finally, they were given a role of keeping families informed and updated regularly. Their role also included memento work and making use of digital technologies to facilitate last conversations between patients and their loved ones. Cygnets were provided with training in communication skills and bereavement work. Their role was intended to supplement and not replace clinical end of life care. At the time of writing, this project is in the process of being evaluated. However, initial anecdotal feedback from the cygnets has been that they have highly valued the opportunity to help support the effort to provide compassionate end of life care and bereavement care during this difficult time. Families, care homes, and ward staff have fed back that it has been reassuring to know that patients have not been alone.

KEY POINTS

- The ability to collaborate across professional boundaries depends not only on the individual members of the team, but on wider organisational structures and

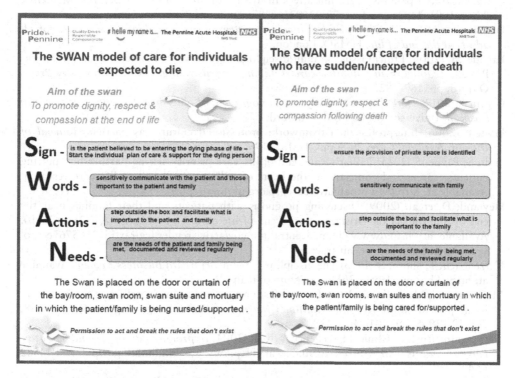

FIGURE 3.1 The "SWAN" model (courtesy of www.pat.nhs.uk)

processes which promote communication and co-ordination of care, to reduce the risk of fragmentation and duplication.

- Tensions between the ideals of collaborative care provision and the realities of clinical care must be addressed.
- Key challenges include balancing the need for expertise whilst maximising continuity of care.
- Effective team-working can be achieved through a focus on collaborative goal-setting in order to benefit patients and carers.

REFERENCES

Barton, A, Mulley, G (2003) History of the development of geriatric medicine in the UK. *Postgraduate Medical Journal*, 229–234; quiz 233–234. doi: 10.1136/pmj.79.930.229

Brogaard, T, et al. (2011) Who is the key worker in palliative home care? *Scandinavian Journal of Primary Health Care*, 29(3), 150–156.

Cousin, G, Schmid Mast, M, Jaunin-Stalder, N (2013) When physician-expressed uncertainty leads to patient dissatisfaction: a gender study. *Medical Education*, 47(9), 923–931. doi: 10.1111/medu.12237

den Herder-van der Eerden, M, van Wijngaarden, J, Payne, S, Preston, N, Linge-Dahl, L, Radbruch, L, Hasselaar, J (2018). Integrated palliative care is about professional networking rather than standardisation of care: a qualitative study with healthcare professionals in

19 integrated palliative care initiatives in five European countries. *Palliative Medicine*, 32(6), 1091–1102. doi: 10.1177/0269216318758194.

Department of Health (2008) *End of life care strategy: promoting high quality care for all adults at the end of life*. HMSO, London.

Farsides, B (2006) Ethical issues in multidisciplinary teams within palliative care, in Speck, P (ed.), *Teamwork in palliative care: fulfilling or frustrating*. Oxford University Press, Oxford, pp. 167–182.

Green, L (2017) *Here there is nobody: an ethnographic of older peoples' end-of-life care in hospital*. University of Bradford: Bradford, UK.

Hall, P (2006) Interprofessional teamwork: professional cultures as barriers. *Journal of Interprofessional Care*, 29(Suppl. 1), 188–196.

Hall, S, Payne, S (2015) Palliative and end of life care priority setting partnership: putting patients, carers and clinicians at the heart of palliative and end of life care research. Available at: http://www.palliativecarepsp.org.uk/finalreport/.

Heyland, D, et al. (2009) Discussing prognosis with patients and their families near the end of life: impact on satisfaction with end-of-life care. *Open Medicine*, 3(2), e101–10. Available at: http://www.pubmedcentral.nih.gov/articlerender.fcgi?artid=2765767&tool =pmcentrez&rendertype=abstract.

Katzenbach, T, Smith, D (1993) The discipline of teams. *Harvard Business Review*. Available at: https://hbr.org/1993/03/the-discipline-of-teams-2.

McDonald, C, McCallin, A (2010) Interprofessional collaboration in palliative nursing: what is the patient-family role? *International Journal of Palliative Nursing*, 16(6), 285–288. doi: 10.12968/ijpn.2010.16.6.48832.

National Institute for Clinical Excellence (NICE) (2004) *Improving supportive and palliative care for adults with cancer*. Available at: http://www.ncbi.nlm.nih.gov/pubmed/14562 664.

National Institute for Clinical Excellence (NICE) (2019) *End of life care for adults: service delivery*.

NHS England (2020) We are the NHS: people plan action for us all, pp. 1–27. Available at: https://www.england.nhs.uk/wp-content/uploads/2020/07/Easy_Read_NHS_People_ Plan-29Jul20.pdf.

Northern Care Alliance (2020) *The SWAN team*. Available at: https://www.pat.nhs.uk/pa tients-and-visitors/swan-model-of-care.htm (accessed 18 May 2020).

O'Brien, M, et al. (2016) Improving end of life care in care homes: an evaluation of the six steps to success programme. *BMC Palliative Care*, 15(53). doi: 10.1186/s12904-016-0123-6

Oishi, A, Murtagh, FEM (2014) The challenges of uncertainty and interprofessional collaboration in palliative care for non-cancer patients in the community: a systematic review of views from patients, carers and health-care professionals. *Palliative Medicine*, 28(9), 1081–1098. doi: 10.1177/0269216314531999

Øvretveit, J (1995) Team decision-making. *Journal of Interprofessional Care*, 9(1), 41–51.

Pattenden J, Mason A, Lewin R. (2013) Collaborative palliative care for advanced heart failure: outcomes and costs from the "Better Together" pilot study. *BMJ Support Palliat Care*. Mar;3(1), 69–76, Epub 2012 Sep 5.

Saunders, C (2001) The evolution of palliative care. *Journal of the Royal Society of Medicine*, 94, 430–432.

Sharp, T, Malyon, A, Barclay, S (2018) GPs' perceptions of advance care planning with frail and older people: a qualitative study. *British Journal of General Practice*, 68(666), e44 LP–e53. doi: 10.3399/bjgp17X694145

Shaw, J, et al. (2016) Interprofessional team building in the palliative home care setting: use of a conceptual framework to inform a pilot evaluation. *Journal of Interprofessional Care*, 30(2), 262–264. doi: 10.3109/13561820.2015.1115395

Thomas, K, et al. (2007) Improving the delivery of palliative care in general practice: an evaluation of the first phase of the Gold Standards Framework. *Palliative Medicinee*, 21(1), 49–53. Available at: http://search.ebscohost.com/login.aspx?direct=true&db=rzh&AN=106022419&site=ehost-live.

Thomas, K, Lobo, B (2011) *Advance care planning in end of life dare*. OUP, Oxford. Available at: https://books.google.com/books?id=CGAk4m0XxY0C&pgis=1.

UK National Palliative and End of Life Care Partnership and National End of Life Care Programme (2015) Ambitions for palliative and end of life care: a national framework for local action 2015–2020. *London* 481, 1–6. Available at: http://eprints.lancs.ac.uk/32387/.

CHAPTER 4

Caring for the person in their world

Collaboration in context

....

Victoria Ali

OUTLINE

Providing care in the person's home can allow the healthcare professional a unique perspective on the person they are caring for, and interaction with their home environment can assist in addressing what is truly important to them at the end of their life. A home (or lack thereof) can give countless clues to the person's lived reality which they may either not immediately share or indeed appreciate exists. A person's home is their metaphorical castle and a place of safety. However, when ill health arises and healthcare needs increase, we risk damaging this by our actions as healthcare professionals. It is important to remember that, as healthcare professionals, we are invited guests into the person's home and as such need to respect their home environment. Accordingly, we need to view ourselves as invited in to be a co-producer of care led by the patient and involving those important to them.

Following a palliative diagnosis, the majority of the person's time, if we get it right, should be spent in their home, yet policy tends to focus upon acute and hospice care at this time. This chapter will focus upon how considering individual patient needs allows a patient-led system of care and how we can facilitate people to remain at home if that is what they wish. Considering this, the language we use may change from questions of preferred place of care to "if you had the right support would you want to die at home and what support would you need to achieve this?"

BACKGROUND: DYING AT HOME

It is important, from the outset, to reflect upon the term "home". The term is used here to refer to wherever a person lives and that the principles of collaborative practice and support can be considered and adapted irrespective of where the person is located. Partly due to the ageing population, care homes, hostels, prisons, secure

DOI: 10.4324/9781351113472-4

mental health settings will all be required, if not already doing so, to provide care to those with palliative care needs and at the end of their life. A majority of people, when asked, express the wish to die at home, however only around 24% do (ONS, 2017). There are assumptions that home may become a "less attractive" option as people deteriorate, however within a systematic review by Gomes et al. (2013), four-fifths of people did not alter their wishes as their illnesses progressed. If the predicted rise of deaths within the United Kingdom occurs as suggested by 2040, there will be a 25.4% increase in the number of people dying within England and Wales (Etkind et al., 2017) and 15.9% in Scotland (Finucane et al., 2019) each year. With an estimated two-thirds of these expected to occur outside of hospital, there is an urgent need for a refocus on the provision of palliative care in the non-hospital setting. The need for effective palliative care within the home environment has never been more pressing.

Within a Cochrane review, Shepperd et al. (2016) identified that provision of home-based care increased the likelihood of a person achieving death at home even when there is sufficient hospice, inpatient care, and primary care provision. Yet the desire, and ability, to die at home is not homogenous across society and key factors have been suggested as affecting this:

- Patients functional status and disease status.
- Preferences and ability to express preference.
- Home care provision being available.
- Intensity of home care provision and support offered based on need.
- Living with relatives.
- Extended family support.
- Availability of hospital beds.

(Gomes and Higginson, 2006)

Having the ability to express a preference, or even simply being asked, has been highlighted as a key issue, and congruence with relatives' wishes was identified as important in ultimately achieving preferred place of death (Gomes and Higginson, 2006). Also identified are inequalities in care access due to underlying condition and poor functional status, and a key function of progressive end of life services should be to afford everyone the same opportunity to meet their preferred place of care and death.

The previous chapters considered challenges relating to transitions between care settings and interdisciplinary working. This chapter will focus upon the challenges of providing individualised patient-centred care at home with a specific focus on addressing inequality in access to healthcare in order to meet individualised needs at the end of life.

CHALLENGES: MAKING THE SERVICE FIT THE PATIENT NOT THE PATIENT FIT THE SERVICE

It must be noted that there is high variability in the configuration of formal care provision at home, depending on which services are commissioned. There are models which involve a multidisciplinary team, some who work more in isolation, hospice at home, and outreach services. Working effectively within a wider multidisciplinary team is essential in providing holistic support at the end of life. However there is no defined standard in how this translates into practice (Payne et al., 2017) or whether these models can be applied to different disease processes (Siouta et al., 2016).

It is important to understand the population demographics at the point of service-level commissioning for palliative and end of life care in order to ensure local needs can be met. However, all too often these services are designed around the needs of pre-existing patients who access the services. Whilst of course this is important, it also a missed opportunity to consider how services can best serve the whole community, and those with unmet needs. Evaluation of services may be based on the achievement of preferred place of care and death, but this will miss out those who did not have the opportunity to access the care provided.

The provision for "hard to reach" groups

The Care and Quality Commission report *A Different Ending* (CQC, 2016) highlighted inequalities in provision of care at end of life, suggesting there are a number of groups whose needs were not well supported or understood. The report identified ten key groups within the briefing, these being:

- People with conditions other than cancer.
- Older people.
- People with dementia.
- People from Black and Minority Ethnic (BME) groups.
- Lesbian, gay, bisexual, or transgender people.
- People with a learning disability.
- People with a mental health condition.
- People who are homeless.
- People who are in secure or detained settings.
- Gypsies and Travellers.

Consider the demographics of the patients within the service you work, are the people in the categories above accurately represented? You may also consider if the referral criteria for the palliative care service you work in or with is inclusive, open to anyone who needs it, and available for all. Yet if you cannot answer definitely answer "yes" to the question above, can we be assured of equity of access into our services?

A term often used to describe these groups is "hard to reach", this term in itself being a problematic descriptor as it suggests an active process being undertaken by people in order to remove themselves from clinical services. This may be the case for some individuals, as is a person's autonomous right, but using this term to describe a group is an unhelpful narrative which needs to be changed. Quite simply our services are not configured in a way to meet the needs of these groups; it is healthcare that is at fault.

SOLUTIONS AND DEVELOPMENTS

A number of practical examples will be given within this chapter to illustrate initiatives and standards that enable the delivery of personalised care.

Case study 1: Providing care based on individual need

Eamon a 62-year-old with acute myeloid leukaemia, he was diagnosed 18 months previously and has received first line chemotherapy. Despite a period of remission the disease has relapsed and he is now receiving palliative rather than curative treatment. He had been attending his local hospital haematology day unit regularly for his full blood count to be checked and to have blood and platelet transfusions when required, around weekly. Recently he has been in hospital more frequently due to infections secondary to bone marrow failure. There are no further anti-cancer treatments available for him and he has already said that he understands that he is dying.

He has a wife who works at a local primary school. She has needed to take time off recently due to Eamon's health and is worried about keeping her job. She also struggles to visit the hospital as she does not drive.

He is asked "What is important to you for your future care?"

He states being with his wife is his priority as he is worried about her health visiting him in hospital and also the financial worries relating to her job. He states he just wants to "make what remains of my life as simple as possible" and "I also want to be at home on the sofa with my dogs as much as I can".

From questioning Eamon, it is clear that his concerns are not health-focused but rather his priorities are the wider social aspects of his life and who he is as a person. Asking *what is important* rather than focussed questioning around preferred place of care will elicit a wider understanding of the essence of the person and what they may want in the future. From Eamon's answers we could infer he would rather be at home. Making this inference, an educated guess, "It sounds from what you have said that you would prefer to be at home if this was possible" would be a useful communication tool to show understanding at this point.

For Eamon to remain at home there are two medical considerations to facilitate this:

1. Managing recurrent infections.
2. Managing symptomatic anaemia.

Firstly, establishing the ceiling of treatment for the infection is required, as this will aid community decision-making about the appropriateness of hospital admission. In this case, considering Eamon's wishes, the ceiling of treatment for infection may be oral antibiotics or intravenous antibiotics at home if this is available.

Haematological malignancies pose a particular challenge for services due to "transfusion tether", essentially that the frequency of transfusions required means that outreach or ambulatory services can be unable to meet the patient's needs and they remain in hospital (Mannis et al., 2016). In this situation, with transfusion as a mainstay of effective symptom management, there may be the perception that the patient is receiving "active" treatment and this can inhibit referral for palliative care support. Early involvement from specialist palliative care services is important, though it is recognised that within haematology this is often challenging and referral may be limited (Howell et al., 2011; Moreno-Alonso et al., 2017; McCaughan et al., 2018). For patients who require transfusion and wish to remain at home there is a role for home blood transfusion services, often incorporated within a community intravenous therapy team, reactive care teams, or embedded with the role of the community nursing service. The person can be transfused regularly at home, eliminating exhausting trips to hospital, with support from a community multidisciplinary team. There is evidence to suggest that this provision can improve quality of life in terms of breathlessness and fatigue management, and prolong life, for many advanced cancers not just haematological malignancies (Payne et al., 2019; Preston et al., 2012).

For people receiving transfusions in day therapy or ambulatory settings, the inability to attend hospital day services due to a reduction in ambulation was deemed an important factor within prognostication and when there may be no further benefit to transfusion. When patients are transfused at home it is important to establish the goals of the treatment and to discuss at the outset that there will be a time when transfusion is no longer appropriate. This is to ensure that the person and those involved in their care are aware that there will be a point where transfusion is no longer providing a clinical benefit and should be discontinued. These pre-emptive discussions are vital to avoid more difficult discussions around withdrawal or continued inappropriate treatment as the person deteriorates.

Case study 2: Symptom management at end of life

Aleena is a 62-year-old woman with end stage heart failure and Chronic Obstructive Pulmonary Disease (COPD). Over the past year she has had increasing admissions to hospital with exacerbations of her COPD requiring management with intravenous antibiotic and steroids. Following her last admission, it was felt that hospital admissions were no longer improving her condition and that the ceiling of treatment for future management could be provided at home and she was discharged home for end of life care. She was previously attending the local hospital ambulatory centre for Intravenous administration of Furosemide 240mg to manage symptoms caused by heart failure. She is now too unwell to travel and is housebound, with her condition deteriorating, and she can only take oral diuretics intermittently. She develops pulmonary oedema if she does not take the full dose of the Furosemide daily. She is aware that she is dying and wishes to remain at home and to be cared for by her daughter. She is reviewed jointly by the Clinical Nurse Specialist in palliative care and community heart failure team who, on assessment, feel that there is a risk of readmission to hospital. They feel that she will become more symptomatic from the pulmonary oedema as she becomes increasingly unable to take the oral medication. She is being cared for by her daughter and she states that these symptoms are already distressing, and she may contact ambulance services. Whilst there is an advance care plan in place, Aleena's wishes may change if her symptom burden becomes intolerable. The decision was made by the multidisciplinary team to convert the oral Furosemide to the subcutaneous route to be delivered over a 24-hour period via a continuous subcutaneous infusion pump and for this to be supported at home.

The case study is chosen in order to encourage the consideration of wider symptom management concerns at end of life, linking back to the ten key aspects of inequality at end of life, for those dying from a disease other than cancer. Local and national policies are being developed to support the use of subcutaneous Furosemide at home at end of life. It is important to be clear with both the multidisciplinary healthcare teams and the patient that the intention of this intervention is to manage symptoms in the end stages of heart failure and reduce the symptom burden of the pulmonary oedema from discontinued oral treatment. Due to this, invasive interventions such as weighing the patient and checking urea and electrolytes is unlikely to alter the management and as such should be avoided. Regular joint reviews with the multidisciplinary team will be required; this may include the general practitioner, clinical nurse specialists in heart failure and palliative care and the district nursing service. Gaining the support of, and collaborating with, local pharmacies is also required to ensure timely access to this medication, as it is unlikely to be stocked routinely within community pharmacies.

Does it always have to be a healthcare professional?

Whilst we have mostly discussed the input and impact of healthcare professionals within this chapter, it would be remiss to not also consider the role of family and friends as informal carers. In fact, I propose that they are a fundamental member of the multidisciplinary team, for without them healthcare professionals would surely struggle to provide any form of effective and safe care at home. I must note, though, that I have witnessed inspiring examples of community nurses taking on this role in the short term, against the odds and at short notice, enabling people to die at home, working above their role and duty. This is not, however, a sustainable or realistic option within current resources in most situations.

The input of informal carers in supporting people to be cared for and to die, if they wish, at home cannot be underestimated. Informal carers may already be involved in the management of symptoms and potentially for a considerable period of time. Healthcare professionals should take care not to disempower carers, who are often better placed to assess the nuances of symptoms as they know the person much better than we could ever hope. For patients in rural areas (and even in urban areas with quicker response times from community nurses) there may be a role for relatives to administer injectable medication to facilitate timely intervention within symptom management. Whilst carers commonly give injections, low-molecular weight heparin and insulin as two examples, additional support for the carer would be required at the end of the patient's life. This includes consideration of how their role in administration of medication may affect their own wellbeing. For example, it is important that the carer understands the intention and effect of the medication (that they are not hastening death), and that they are not responsible if symptoms are not adequately managed, so that this does not have a lasting impact on their bereavement process. At present, we have a limited understanding of the impact on carers of administering injectable medications, so it is important that further research informs practice (Bowers et al., 2018). An example of how this can be supported is given by Lee et al. (2016) who developed a policy for administration of injectable medication by carers.

ADDRESSING INEQUALITIES

A Marie Curie (2016) commissioned report highlighted the work required in addressing inequalities in access to care at end of life and improving the experience in relation to the LGBTQ+ community. They identified six key areas:

1) Anticipated discrimination within healthcare systems where needs may be poorly understood.
2) Inequality in access to religious and spiritual care.
3) Assumptions about gender identity and family structure.
4) Recognition of the individual's support structure and next of kin as a non-relative.
5) Unsupported grief and bereavement.
6) Increased impact on informal carers due to lack of formal support.

A study by Stonewall (2015) found that only 57% of health and social care practitioners in patient-facing roles felt that sexual orientation was relevant to a person's health and social care needs. If healthcare professionals do not consider sexual orientation as a relevant aspect of care, they will fail in the provision of holistic care, and perpetuate discrimination, making aspects of personal identity invisible. The LGBTQ+ community has also identified a lack of engagement from healthcare professionals with partners, spouses, and those important to them. This may indicate a lack of understanding about who and what may be important to the person and possible assumptions that family structures are not present. However, we do not know unless we ask. Do not avoid having advance care planning discussions for fear, be conscious that relationship status or gender identity may not be known to everyone, and careful navigation of this may be required. The use of neutral questioning is required, in order to remove assumptions and judgement calls. Consider asking everyone the same question, simply "who are the important people in your life?".

Both the CQC report (2016) and the Marie Curie report (2016) recognise that underrepresentation of minority groups within end of life care research means that their needs have not been transferred into policy. This is something being addressed by researchers by Manchester Metropolitan University for people who misuse substances (Witham et al., 2019). This collaborative project between academics, palliative care services, and addiction services has developed key policy standards in order to ensure the needs of this group do not continue to be marginalised. The key points raised within the report relate to reducing stigma and stereotyping, developing national policy to support co-existing services, and ensuring an accessible care environment. It is acknowledged that joint working across substance use services, palliative care, and primary care is required to support patients and those important to them. Appropriate education and training also need to be in place for all healthcare staff to ensure that the range of patient needs are understood across care boundaries. Whilst the genesis of this project was to improve the experience of those with a history of substance misuse who are at the end of life, it is clear that this is not the only population that is currently underserved. Other vulnerable groups, including the homeless population and those with mental health issues, also have complex needs that require the support of a range of health services.

The art of reflection is essential in order to identify any unconscious biases which may affect holistic care provision within these identified groups. The use of the word "assumptions" in this section is also important and purposeful; we should not make assumptions about people, their beliefs, and what may or may not be important to them. This an ethical principle which should run though our care provision irrespective of who we are providing care for.

Case study 3: Location as a limitation to care provision

John is a 69-year-old male who has been cared for within a maximum-security mental health unit for the past ten years. He has been diagnosed with Parkinson's disease, he is becoming increasingly frail and has been experiencing an increased symptom burden over the past two months. The nurse from the unit contacts the community palliative care team to discuss the care of the patient. They have access to a GP clinic once a week but they are worried about how they may be able to provide the care he needs as his condition deteriorates. They are also unsure if there may be needs that are already unmet due to the mental health focus of the unit. The palliative care service had not provided care in this environment before and the services were not within the same provider organisation. From the discussions it was clear that the patient's needs were urgent and as such a service level agreement to provide support was required.

The main ethical concern for both services, and the starting point for planning, is that the patient has the right to access the same level of care irrespective of where is classed as home. As there is not current access to palliative care provision, the first step is to ensure that the management team in both provider organisations support the assessment and delivery of care in the secure setting. This can be mitigated with a service level agreement across organisations to ensure clear governance structures are in place outlining the roles and responsibilities of staff across both provider organisations and escalation and support plans for healthcare staff delivering care.

The primary consideration, however, should not be different from the general principles of good palliative care: what is the person's preferred place of care and death? Does the patient have capacity to be involved in this discussion, and is it safe for them to be cared for in an alternative care environment? If the person is increasingly physically frail due to their deteriorating condition, are they a physical risk to themselves or others? If this is no longer a consideration then can discharge be planned in order for them to die where they choose? It may be that they wish to remain where they are, as a place of safety, and for some patients there may be no other safe option for them.

Where collaboration across organisations is required, staff training needs must also be addressed (Witham et al., 2019). In this case, training for mental health staff on expected disease trajectory and symptom management was valuable. Reciprocal training for physical health staff was also given, in order to understand the impact of the enduring mental health condition and the care environment, and this fed into the care planning process. In terms of practical provision there are also a number of considerations dependent upon the structure of the services involved. For example, can the mental health service directly contact a palliative care clinician for advice and is there out-of-hours support for the unit and how, and by whom, will this be delivered? Do staff on the unit feel confident to administer injectable medication for symptom management or is this better placed with the community physical health services as "inreach" into the unit? If the latter is the case then the practicalities of entering the secure setting also need to be considered. Consideration was also given to the time taken to enter into the unit with security checks, especially out-of-hours when there are reduced numbers of community staff.

Although this case is in a secure mental health setting, the practical issues are similar when addressing the needs of those at the end of life in prisons. For further reading around this see Turner and Peacock (2017) and *Dying Well in Custody Charter* linked to the palliative care ambitions document (Ambitions for Palliative and End of Life Care 2018).

This leads back to the initial thoughts that care, irrespective of where is home, has the same foundation. I could argue that the aspects considered within this chapter are just good planning, timely access to medication, training staff to provide care, assessing risk, and overall ensuring access to care for the patient in the right place for them. The challenge for us, as healthcare professionals, is not seeing the boundaries and barriers to our services. I would argue that it is our duty of care as healthcare professionals, whilst ensuring patient safety, to push the boundaries of services to shape them around our patients based on their needs.

KEY POINTS

- The importance of proactive care planning based on individualised patient need.
- What is it about the needs of people who are less likely to die in their home environment that means this does not happen? Understanding this allows us to develop care provision to meet the needs of all in society.
- Engaging these groups in designing services that are truly inclusive: do not assume you are inclusive if you have never asked.
- Remember the key questions: "What do I need to know about you in order to be able to care for you?"
- "Would you want to die at home and what support would you need to achieve this?"

REFERENCES

Ambitions for Palliative and End of Life Care (2018) *Dying well in custody charter*. http://end oflifecareambitions.org.uk/tag/prisons/

Bowers, B, Ryan, R, Kuhn, I, Barclay, S (2018) Anticipatory prescribing of injectable medications for adults at the end of life in the community: a systematic literature review and narrative synthesis. *Palliative Medicine*, 33, 160–177.

Care and Quality Commission (2016) *A different ending: addressing inequalities in end of life care*. CQC, London.

Etkind, SN, Bone, AE, Gomes, B, Lovell, N, Evans, CJ, Higginson, IJ, Murtaggh, FEM (2017) How many people will need palliative care in 2040? Past trends, future projections and implications for services. *BMC Medicine*, 15, 102–110.

Finucane, AM, Bone, AE, Evans, CJ, Gomes, B, Meade, R, Higginson, IJ, Murray, SA (2019) The impact of population ageing on end-of-life care in Scotland: projections of place of death and recommendations for future service provision. *BMC Palliative Care*, 18, 112–111.

Gomes, B, Calanzani, N, Curiale, V, McCrone, P, Higginson, IJ (2013) Effectiveness and cost-effectiveness of home palliative care services for adults with advanced illness and their caregivers. *The Cochrane Database of Systematic Reviews*, 6(6), CD007760.

Gomes, B, Higginson, IJ (2006) Factors influencing death at home in terminally ill patients with cancer: systematic review. *BMJ*, 332, 515–521.

Howell, DA, Shellens, R, Roman, E, Garry, AC, Patmore, R, Howard, MR (2011) Haematological malignancy: are patients appropriately referred for specialist palliative and hospice care? A systematic review and meta-analysis of published data. *Palliative Medicine*, 25, 630–641.

Lee, L, Howard, K, Wilkinson, L, Kern, C, Hall, S (2016) Developing a policy to empower informal carers to administer subcutaneous medication in community palliative care; a feasibility project. *International Journal of Palliative Nursing*, 22, 369–378.

Mannis, GN, McNey, LM, Gupta, NK, Gross, DM (2016) The transfusion tether: bridging the gap between end-stage hematologic malignancies and optimal end-of-life care. *American Journal of Hematology*, 91, 364–365.

Marie Curie (2016) Hiding who I am: the reality of end of life care for LGBT people. Available at: https://www.mariecurie.org.uk/globalassets/media/documents/policy/policy-publica tions/june-2016/reality-end-of-life-care-lgbt-people.pdf

McCaughan, D, Roman, E, Smith, AG, Garry, AC, Johnston, MJ, Patmore, RD, Howard, MR, Howell, DA (2018) Palliative care specialists' perceptions concerning referral of haematology patients to their services: findings from a qualitative study. *BMC Palliative Care*, 17, 33.

Moreno-Alonso, D, Porta-Sales, J, Monforte-Royo, C, Trelis-Navarro, J, Sureda-Balarí, A, Fernández De Sevilla-Ribosa, A (2017) Palliative care in patients with haematological neoplasms: an integrative systematic review. *Palliative Medicine*, 32, 79–105.

Office of National Statistics (2017) *Death by place of occurrence 2016*. Edited by Office of National Statistics. London.

Payne, S, Eastham, R, Hughes, S, Varey, S, Hasselaar, J, Preston, N (2017) Enhancing integrated palliative care: what models are appropriate? A cross-case analysis. *BMC Palliative Care*, 16, 64–66.

Payne, S, Hughes, S, Wilkinson, J, Hasselaar, J, Preston, N (2019) Recommendations on priorities for integrated palliative care: transparent expert consultation with international leaders for the InSuP-C project. *BMC Palliative Care*, 18, 32–38.

Preston, NJ, Hurlow, A, Brine, J, Bennett, MI (2012) Blood transfusions for anaemia in patients with advanced cancer. *The Cochrane Database of Systematic Reviews*, 2012, CD009007.

Shepperd, S, Gonçalves-Bradley, DC, Straus, SE, Wee, B (2016) Hospital at home: home-based end-of-life care. *Cochrane Database of Systematic Reviews*, 2016, CD009231.

Siouta, N, Van Beek, K, Van Der Eerden, ME, Preston, N, Hasselaar, JG, Hughes, S, Garralda, E, Centeno, C, Csikos, A, Groot, M, Radbruch, L, Payne, S, Menten, J (2016) Integrated palliative care in Europe: a qualitative systematic literature review of empirically-tested models in cancer and chronic disease. *BMC Palliative Care*, 15, 56.

Stonewall (2015) Unhealthy attitudes: the treatment of LGBT people within health and social care services. https://www.stonewall.org.uk/our-work/campaigns/unhealthy-attitudes

Turner, M, Peacock, M (2017) Palliative care in UK prisons. *Journal of Corrective Health Care*, 23, 56–65.

Witham, G, Galvani, S, Peacock, M (2019) End of life care for people with alcohol and drug problems: findings from a rapid evidence assessment. *Health & Social Care in the Community*, 27, e637–e650.

CHAPTER 5

Systems within systems

Collaboration with the family

....

Linda McEnhill and Patricia McCrossan

OUTLINE

Systems theory provides a framework for understanding collaboration between formal and informal systems. This chapter focuses on working with families but has implications for collaboration generally within palliative care.

BACKGROUND

As has been indicated in the opening chapter, palliative care is essentially a collaborative activity, one which draws the expertise of all relevant professions together for the good of the patient, often thereby achieving greater positive outcomes than were possible if only single disciplines and professionals were acting on the patient's behalf.

However, there is another element of collaboration which is integral to palliative care, and that is collaboration with the family. From the inception of palliative care, a defining principle is the assertion that: "The dying person and those who matter to that person [the family] are the unit of care" (National Council for Hospice and Specialist Palliative Care Services, 1995).

The logic of this approach is inescapable: a commitment to a holistic perspective of the patient, and the resulting model of care affirms that "...people should not be viewed as isolated units but always in a context, in a particular set of relationships in which they operate at any given time" (Preston-Shoot and Agass, 1990, p. 53). In practice, as in theory, the family continues to constitute the foundational set of relationships for the patient. Consequently, often the greatest distress that a patient will experience is not so much related to the dying process but to the existential sadness of failed or complex familial relationships. The family is the stage on which our greatest successes and/or failures are played out and thus at the end of life attracts great energy and focus.

So too for each family member, individually and collectively, as they face the cumulative losses and ultimate bereavement of their kin person, the breaking of fundamental

DOI: 10.4324/9781351113472-5

attachments, loss of shared memories, and ways of being. It is no surprise then that one of the ways of conceiving of bereavement is the loss of the reflection of ourselves as we were in relationship with the person who has died, i.e. the big or little (albeit now adult) sister, the daughter, father, mother. No surprise either that even deeply fractured families may try to reunite around blood bonds at the end of life with all the consequent achievements, reconciliations, bitter disappointments, and furious arguments this may bring. The family is thus the "unit of care" in the sense of all those who comprise the need for care but also the greatest resource for deep, emotional support which facilitates acceptable meanings in even the worst of circumstances.

SYSTEMS MODEL: DEVELOPMENT, MAIN FEATURES, AND APPLICATION

From the 1950s, systemic models began to be developed adding greater dimension to therapeutic relationships which had previously been limited to dyadic, problem saturated client/therapist engagements, often looking no further than pathologising the behaviour of the client. In systemic thinking, families are not just a group of individuals but rather are interdependent members of established social systems with roles, alliances, boundaries, and power. The inherent systems and subsystems develop cyclical patterns and sequences of behaviour that appear to enable them to achieve or return to a level of homeostasis (Von Bertalanffy, 1968).

Building on these principles, Salvador Minuchin developed the structural, systemic concept of family therapy. Subsequent socio-political and feminist critiques of this model, particularly its application of neutrality to issues of power, have led to reformation of the model into the Post Milan approach (Brown, 2010). It extended structural systemic principles by including hypothesising, curiosity, circularity, and neutrality as tools to be utilised in interviewing families to arrive at an effective understanding of the family system. These were revolutionary in seeking to undermine or "cast off" the previous therapeutic models which gave primacy to the personal qualities of the therapist such as intuition, charisma, and concern.

Where traditional, structural family therapy establishes the professional in a first order or expert position, Post Milan approaches enable the professional to take a second order position within the family system (Palazzoli et al., 1980). This encourages the family to become curious and question each other, prompting and enabling them to produce helpful, meaningful information about how they interact and understand each other. As the family system evolves, previously established coping mechanisms may no longer be effective in restoring balance and meaning. Introducing curiosity, hypothesis, neutrality, and circular questioning can support a family to safely self-regulate and reconstruct new meaning, as a result of self-correcting feedback (Burnham, 1988), as will be demonstrated in the case study later in the chapter.

SYSTEMIC THINKING IN PALLIATIVE CARE

Families however are complex entities. Any particular family may appear to be an unintelligible maze of alliances and coalitions with cultures which seem illogical and impenetrable to the "outsider". This is all exacerbated by closed or barely permeable family boundaries that frustrate even the most skilled and experienced palliative care professional, who may simultaneously have productive interactions with individual family members but still be unable to engage the family in its entirety to good effect. The importance of being able to do so however cannot be overestimated, particularly in the light of Kissane and Bloch's research which indicates that "dysfunctional" family relationships and communication may predispose to complex bereavement reactions after the death of the patient (Kissane and Bloch, 2002).

Those professionals who are trained in systemic interventions, prioritising relationships over individuals, have unique assets to offer in palliative care. Traditionally the work of palliative care social workers, who are inherently context driven, and more recently family therapists, they are able to offer focussed interventions with an emphasis on helping the family to do what "they" do best in terms of how they negotiate and resolve the various challenges of life. They bring perspectives which are almost hidden from individually focussed theorists and practitioners both on the nature of families and of organisations (such as hospices) as systems.

The work of the late Frances Sheldon deserves note in this section. As one of the early palliative care social workers she did much to enhance expertise in psychosocial care, most particularly in the development of the Masters in Psychosocial Palliative Care based at Southampton University. Extending the, until then, almost unique skillset of the systemically trained palliative care social worker to other professionals, she explicated for many Cicely Saunders' concept of "total pain". Sheldon reiterates the primacy of the family as the "unit of care"; she says:

A holistic view necessarily takes into account the relationships of the dying person... based on a systemic view of relationships which recognises that each individual affects, and is affected by, those closest to them. This does not mean that the views of relatives will be weighted more heavily than those of the dying person, but that the interdependence of all parties is understood. The pain of the family is different but may be as great, sometimes greater than that of the dying person.

(Sheldon 1997, p. 9)

It is important to remember that some members of the "unit of care" will be children or young people. Only in the last two decades or so have the needs of children and young people facing the challenges of serious illness or death in the family been recognised. Prior to this they were relatively neglected and even hospice support services were rarely adapted to meet the cognitive and experiential needs of these young people. This is despite swathes of evidence demonstrating that unresolved childhood grief predisposes to a range of negative impacts including adult depression, offending behaviour, and reduced life chances. The work of the Childhood Bereavement Network (see www.childhoodbereavementnetwork.org.uk) has revolutionised how society in general, and hospices in particular, understand the needs of these young people. In terms of systemic approaches, the models are perhaps less well developed with regard to young people's ability to influence the system rather than being seen as purely passively influenced by it. The case study below explicates why this is a partial understanding of what roles children and young people play within the family system and its ability to rewrite the family script to take account of the new environment engendered by serious illness, death, and bereavement.

KEY SYSTEMIC PRINCIPLES IN COLLABORATING WITH PATIENTS AND FAMILIES IN PALLIATIVE CARE

Collaboration between multidisciplinary professionals is an essential and valued component of palliative care. Indeed, the team of professionals supporting the dying, and those significant to them, is ever expanding, with everyone eager to contribute their own specific element of "expertise". Whilst dying may have become less medicalised, the question is whether that has been substituted by it becoming professionalised (Clark, 2002), e.g. can we only hope to achieve a "good death" with a team of expert professionals embracing us and leading the way? As indicated above, relational factors significantly influence how people adapt and cope with their emotional response to death and dying, and collaborative engagement facilitates effective coping mechanisms (Zaider, Kissane, 2009). Early, consistent intervention can be crucial in supporting families to cope with the stress and uncertainty brought by illness and attempts to deal with it (Rolland, 2005).

As practitioners we need to consider how often we authentically recognise the people we support as experts and engage in meaningful collaboration with them. Can we truly work in collaboration when we generally acknowledge and respond to people as "patients", "carers", and "loved ones"? Working in partnership with people and understanding what is important to them, allowing them to define the pace and level of engagement, may feel like a challenge initially, but it contributes to a solid foundation for a meaningful partnership.

Within systemic practice, although concepts of hypothesis, circularity, neutrality, and curiosity were initially developed in the 1980s (Selvini et al., 1980), they are still relevant to practice today. They can be utilised to support practitioners to work collaboratively with families and introduce alternative approaches for them to change the way they understand and interact with each other. We outline these principles briefly below.

Hypothesis: The practitioner's role is to formulate hypotheses to generate a potential explanation that aids understanding of relational interaction and function between all members of the family system. Hypotheses are a useful starting point to inform assessment and analysis and should be constantly tested for usefulness in understanding systemic connections, relationships, behaviours, and beliefs, e.g. adults make choices or behave in ways they explain as "protecting the children", but are they rather protecting themselves? Studies indicate that 65% of families display patterns of unhelpful communication when someone is dying and link this to trying to avoid distress and maintain hope (Zhang, Siminoff, 2003).

Testing hypotheses for "usefulness not truthfulness" (Dallas and Draper, 2015) helps the practitioner to avoid becoming wedded to a hypothesis and then only searching for information which will confirm their hypothesis was correct. The information gained in testing a "false" hypothesis generates the formation of another hypothesis which might prove more useful. Multiple hypotheses can be creatively considered to generate ideas and hope.

Circularity: This invites a family to explore the circularity of their interaction to formulate new information, views, and responses (Nelson et al., 1986). Instead of speaking for themselves they are asked to comment on their perceptions of the behaviour and connections of others. This can create a powerful foundation to support transition (Cecchin, 1987).

Neutrality: The professional isn't indifferent or inactive but listens without prejudice and avoids presenting any judgement, labelling of behaviours, or suggestions about how the family should behave. If a family argue, they might ask the family, "who appears to enjoy the arguments the most?" or "who would miss the arguing if it ceased?" to help the family explore and understand why arguments had become part of their interaction. This can also generate families to find their own solutions (Goldenberg & Goldenberg, 1995).

Circularity and neutrality are intimately interlinked as inviting family members to comment on the relationships between each other can enable the professional to remain neutral and thereby form alliances with each member of the family system. It neutralises power struggles, privileged relationships, blaming, and pathologising. Circular questions can be asked of one individual to comment on the relationship or behaviour of others and then others may be asked if they agree (Nelson et al., 1986).

Curiosity: Working in collaboration with some families may require less direct multidisciplinary involvement. For example, recognising a generational family script embedded in the culture of the armed forces and described by the family as constantly relocating, not showing emotion, and having few close friendships, was a vital part of developing meaningful engagement in the family described in the case study below (Byng-Hall, 1998).

Case study

I met Joan in my role as hospice social worker. Joan was a 44-year-old, white, British woman, who worked as a sports teacher. She was diagnosed with metastatic breast cancer 4 years previously, developing extensive disease in her lungs, liver and bones. She had chemotherapy and radiotherapy and experienced symptoms of pain, nausea, fatigue and reduced mobility. Joan was strong, determined and very private. She attended the hospice day unit to access acupuncture and to see a doctor for medication reviews to manage her symptoms. She was polite and smiled a lot but kept herself to herself and her attendance was spasmodic.

I later met her husband Ron, who had given up work to become her full-time carer, as he considered agency carers were "not good enough and Joan needs the best". Ron had spent most of his adult life in the armed forces and this was very important to him. Their situation had an impact on their finances, and they asked to meet me to assess whether they might be entitled to any welfare benefits or grants to maximise their income.

They were friendly but appeared uncomfortable and restricted engagement to basic information sharing. They had a daughter and two sons, aged 15–20 years old, who lived with them, but hadn't been told anything about Joan's illness other than she had cancer and was receiving treatment. They were relieved their children didn't ask questions and believed this indicated they were comfortable with the explanation given and would only be distressed if they knew more. Their 15-year-old son had developed behavioural issues that were raising concerns at school and he was becoming argumentative and destructive. His parents suggested that this was typical teenage behaviour and would pass.

I became totally intrigued and curious about their family system but recognised that Joan and Ron needed time to develop trust and define the pace of our engagement.

I met their daughter, Janet (20), and sons Oliver (18) and Dan (15), during Joan's first and subsequent admissions to the Inpatient unit for symptom control, and respite from what was often portrayed as a lively, noisy, chaotic home. Joan opened up and told me more about their family:

Janet was in the process of joining the police, which made them very proud parents.

Oliver was creative and imaginative and studying art at university. Joan felt he was misunderstood and isolated from his dad and siblings.

Dan was still at school, sporty, charming and engaging. He could become very angry and aggressive and had broken windows and furniture at home. When this happened Ron held him in a bear hug, until he calmed down.

Joan's family did not live locally, she was close to her father but not her mother. Her brother was in the armed forces and her sister did not visit much but they had frequent telephone contact. Joan felt her family tolerated Ron, but he often fell out with them. I was never aware of any friends visiting her.

All was going to their plan, until Joan's cancer infiltrated her bone marrow and it was time to share her prognosis of weeks, with their children. They asked me to join them and Joan insisted she would break the news. Dan ran out of the room, followed by his dad, and Joan, who was bedbound, and I were left to console the others who were crying, but not speaking. When Dan and Ron returned to the room it was agreed to have a family discussion.

Having trained as a systemic practitioner I considered how I might get to know the family and formulate useful hypotheses to help my understanding, including:

Ron's relationship with Oliver. How did Ron's military background relate to a son who had dyed his hair, didn't like sport and enjoyed art?

Was Dan's aggressive, destructive behaviour a means of getting a hug?

What insight did the children really have, in an age where information is easily accessed online?

Circular questions were used to support the family to talk and provide feedback about how they perceived relationships and behaviour. They were able to start exploring what needed to change. I was pleasantly surprised how quickly the family embraced and utilised the process of circularity and I recognised that investing the time and energy to get to know them as individuals and part of a family system enabled me to gain the trust required to enable them to feel "secure enough to improvise".

The following are examples of circular questions utilised in the family discussions:

Q: "Janet, what needs to change within the way your parents relate to their children?"
R: "They need to be honest with us."
All the children agreed, and Joan and Ron acknowledged this, and the family discussed how this might be achieved.
Joan shared her concern for Oliver, as she was "the only one who got him".
Q: "How does your dad/Ron show Oliver he cares about him?"
Q: "How do you know when Daniel is upset?"
Q: "How does your dad behave when he is worried?"
Q: "What is the biggest worry for Joan/this family?" – prompted open discussion about Joan dying and her concerns about how they would cope.

Shortly after the meeting Dan asked to meet with me. He produced a letter he had written to his mother shortly after she was initially diagnosed. He apologised for causing her cancer, as he had been told in a science lesson that stress was the main cause of cancer. He considered he had starting misbehaving months before the diagnosis. Dan was very distressed and asked me to share the letter with his mother. I reassured him that he had not caused his mum's cancer and offered to arrange for him to meet with our Medical Director, but he said he accepted my reassurance. He asked me to stay with Joan whilst she read his letter then he would meet with her. Joan was saddened but met with Dan to reassure him. The family subsequently noticed a remarkable change in Dan's behaviour, and he appeared calmer and more open.

After the first meeting Ron told me that each of their sons had approached him that evening and produced readings and music suggestions for Joan's funeral. They had not spoken to each other but had all prepared something several months earlier.

At the request of the family we had short daily meetings and I was increasingly able to step back as their dialogue with each other became naturally circular and more open and honest. They talked about their shared worry of how they would cope after Joan's death and she acknowledged she only wanted Ron with her when she died. The children agreed and suggested that their maternal aunt move in with them whilst Ron remained at the hospice. Oliver started spending more time with his siblings and Ron made a particular effort with him.

Joan died two weeks later, at the hospice and Ron was with her. Her funeral was a celebration of her life and Ron and her sons were actively involved. Ron accessed bereavement support from the hospice and Dan from a local voluntary bereavement support service. Janet did not want to access support and Oliver received support from a peer group at college.

RECOMMENDATIONS FOR FUTURE DEVELOPMENTS
IN SYSTEMIC PRACTICE IN PALLIATIVE CARE

Death and dying understandably generate levels of distress within family systems but currently this is predominantly explored and measured only on an individual basis, often using different assessment models for the patient and other family members. There are three areas for development which would greatly enhance the practice of staff accompanying the experience and functioning of individuals and families facing the challenges of serious ill health, dying, and bereavement. These are:

Enhancing the multiprofessional team's understanding of systemic perspectives and tools

Developing the understanding of the palliative care patient within the concept of a family system would significantly enhance the effectiveness of therapeutic interventions offered to the patient and to the family as the "unit of care". Training the whole multiprofessional team in the utilisation of tools traditionally only used by social workers or systemic therapists, e.g. Ecomaps, would ensure a shared understanding focussing on the strengths of families to meet current challenges through their inherent cohesiveness, expressiveness, and ways of managing conflict. Ecomaps (Hartman, 1978) provide a visual representation of the family and social networks relevant to the individual. As demographics have continued to change over the decades, many people have less contact and attachment to their families and their most meaningful relationships are established on a social or community level. The two concepts can also be merged into an ecogram which can represent a clear, concise, systemic visual image that can be referred to and understood by all. Families, including children, can become involved in compiling any of the tools utilised.

Developing tiered approaches to the assessment and management of distress

The current models of emotional support pre and post bereavement within palliative care remain predominantly dyadic. This is perhaps best evidenced in the regular "family" meetings which tend to focus on discharge planning and medical updates, effectively limiting opportunities to enable the family system to explore their collective, interactive response. It is increasingly clear that if we wish to enhance bereavement outcomes for those family members left behind that there is need for a much more sophisticated understanding of the family system and models of care which result from this.

It is also widely recognised that distress is multi-dimensional and there are several assessment tools to measure individual response, but research relating to collective, systemic responses is limited. Research varies regarding which aspect of distress should be measured, how it is conceptualised, its inter-relational influences and how distress impacts as it reverberates within the system. Carolan, Smith and Forbat (2015) suggest a tiered approach that may initially explore individual concepts of distress and gradually develop interactions to facilitate the individual members of the system to consider their collective understanding, relational function, and response to distress; this perspective is clearly potentially of great value.

Resilience and associated strength or assets-based perspectives

The family as a system may seem to be impenetrable to the external professional and especially at a time when the perceived threat of serious illness and bereavement causes family members to bond ever more closely together and (perhaps unintentionally) exclude any who do not belong. However, it is important to remember that whilst every system has a homeostatic tendency to maintain the status quo it also has the potential for change and an inherent capacity to evolve and transform itself.

It would be useful for multiprofessional palliative care teams to explore how current assets-based philosophies may be aligned with systemic understandings of patients and families (both adults and children) facing the challenges of serious illness, dying, and bereavement and to reconsider "resilience" not only as an individual characteristic but one which is either inherent in, or can be facilitated within, family systems. Effective support for family resilience will enable the finite resources of psychosocial palliative care to target the family and individuals within it who are, perhaps temporarily, struggling to face the ultimate challenges of death, dying, and bereavement (Zaider & Kissane, 2007).

KEY POINTS

- Every individual patient needs to be considered within the context of their relevant family networks or systems.
- The family is the foundational system of the individual and unresolved relational issues within it may complicate the dying process for the patient and the grieving process of their significant others.
- Systemic models of care offer particular insights and specific tools by which to engage with the family, facilitating it to use its inherent resilience, unique strengths, and assets to manage the challenges presented at this stage of its evolution.
- Training all members of the multiprofessional team in systemic assessment and interventions enables more effective partnerships between each member of the family and the family as a whole.
- Effective targeting of finite psychosocial resources to those families who most need support will enable them to express their resilience in the face of the ultimate challenges of dying and bereavement.

REFERENCES

Brown, JM (2010) The Milan principles of hypothesising, circularity and neutrality in dialogical family therapy: extinction, evolution, eviction... or emergence? *The Australian and New Zealand Journal of Family Therapy*, 31(3), 248–265.

Burnham, JB (1988) *Family therapy*. Routledge, New York and London.

Byng-Hall, J (1998) *Rewriting family scripts, improvisation and systems change*. Guildford Press, London.

Carolan, CM, Smith, A, Forbat, L (2015) Conceptualising psychological distress in families in palliative care: findings from a systemic review. *Palliative Medicine*, 29(7), 605–632.

Cecchin, MD (1987) Hypothesising, circularity and neutrality revisited: an invitation to curiosity. *Family Process*, 26(4), 405–413.

Clark, D (2002) Between hope and acceptance: the medicalisation of dying. *British Medical Journal*, 324(7350), 1391.

Dallos, R, Draper, R (2015) *An introduction to family therapy: systemic theory and practice*, 4th ed. Open University Press, London.

Goldenberg, I, Goldenberg, H (1995) *Family therapy - an overview*, 4th ed. USA Brooks/Cole, London.

Hartman, A (1978) Diagrammatic assessment of family relationships. *Social Casework*, 59(8), 456–476.

Kissane, DW, Bloch, S (2002) *Family focused grief therapy: a model of family-centred care during palliative care and bereavement*. Open University Press, Buckingham and Philadelphia.

National Council for Hospice and Specialist Palliative Care Services (NCHSPCS) (1995) *Principles of palliative care*.

Nelson, TS, Fleuridas, C, Rosenthal, DM (1986) The evolution of circular questions: training family therapists. *Journal of Marital and Family Therapy*, 12(2), 113–127.

Palazzoli, MS, Boscolo, L, Cecchin, G, Prata, G (1980) The problem of the referring person. *Journal of Marital and Family Therapy*, 6: 3–9.

Preston-Shoot, M, Agass, D (1990) *Making sense of social work: psychodynamics, system and practice*. Macmillan Press Ltd, London.

Rolland, JS (2005) Cancer and the family: an integrative model. *Cancer*, 14(11) Supplement, 2584–2595.

Selvini, MP, Boscolo, L, Cecchin, G, Prata, G (1980) Hypothesising, circularity, neutrality: three guidelines for the conductor of the session. *Family Process*, 19(1), 3–12.

Sheldon, F. (1997) *Psychosocial palliative care: good practice in the care of the dying and bereaved*. Stanley Thornes Publishers Ltd, Cheltenham.

Von Bertalanffy, L (1968) *General system theory*. Penguin, New York and London.

Zaider, T, Kissane, D (2007) *Resilient families*. In: Monroe, B, Oliviere, D (eds.), *Resilience in palliative care. Achievement in adversity*. Oxford University Press, Oxford.

Zaider, T, Kissane, D (2009) The assessment and management of family distress during palliative care. *Current Opinion in Supportive and Palliative Care*, 3, 67–71.

Zhang, AY, Siminoff, LA (2003) Silence and cancer: why do families and patients fail to communicate? *Health Communication*, 15(4), 415–429.

CHAPTER 6

Building bridges

Collaboration between organisations

....

Manjula Patel

OUTLINE

This chapter describes a novel and successful partnership between a NHS specialist palliative care service and a third sector organisation that delivered two palliative care services for seamless care and support. It will outline the features of the partnership that provided an integrated approach, plus two case studies of how the collaboration in practice impacted on individual care and discuss factors that promote and hinder a collaborative approach.

BACKGROUND: NATIONAL AND LOCAL CONTEXT

At the turn of the century, a major re-organisation of the NHS saw the formation of Primary Care Groups (PCGs); their role was to improve the health of the local population and address health inequalities. A few years later, the PCGs transferred to Primary Care Trusts (PCTs) with greater financial control. There was an emphasis on innovation and partnerships with local authority social care and voluntary sector organisations to develop and deliver local health promoting services (Abbott & Banks-Smith, 2001).

There was a focus on removing the barriers between health and social care to be co-designed around the individual needs rather than the other way round. With an emphasis on integration between community healthcare and social care to enable professionals from different organisations to work together to deliver seamless care. The principle of person-centred care was at the heart of integrated care with all professionals working to achieve the same goal (Lloyd & Wait, 2005).

The Metropolitan Borough of Sandwell is made up of six towns with a population of approximately 300,000; it is one of the urban boroughs that make up the Black Country – a conurbation of the West Midlands. The six towns were twinned to form three PCGs/PCTs before they all merged to become Sandwell PCT.

DOI: 10.4324/9781351113472-6

Historically the area was at the heart of the industrial revolution and the main employment for the population was in heavy industry. It is ranked as 12th most deprived out of the total of 326 local authorities (Department for Communities and Local Government, 2011), with higher than average incidence of many of the major illnesses, and life expectancy continues to be lower than the national average.

Mostly, hospices have been established and are maintained in areas where there is successful public fundraising (Winslow & Meldrum, 2013), hence in a deprived area like Sandwell there has never been an in-patient hospice. The borough has one hospital Trust that provides community health services and the local authority provides social care, but specialist treatment centres such as radiotherapy are in neighbouring boroughs and in-patient specialist palliative care provision is spot purchased from several different hospices settings in neighbouring boroughs.

THIRD SECTOR COMMUNITY HEALTH ORGANISATION

Murray Hall Community Trust is a local charity based in Sandwell, established in 1994 to respond to the inequalities that negatively impact peoples' lives, with a social model of health. Recognising the wider determinants of health, the charity aim is to improve the health and wellbeing of the local population, through community development approaches. At the time the charity was formed there was an emphasis for local PCGs to innovate and develop new partnerships for service delivery. Hence, Sandwell PCG formed a working partnership with Murray Hall to provide health promoting initiatives.

The ambitious NHS plan (Department of Health, 2000) brought significant investment to modernise the NHS and transform patient care. It supported new initiatives in cancer care to not only improve cancer diagnosis, treatment, and waiting times but to also to address the entrenched inequalities of cancer survival within deprived communities where mortality was higher than the national average.

Soon after the NHS Plan (Department of Health, 2000) was published, lottery funding was made available to support the inequalities in cancer care. At the time, Murray Hall consulted with local people and they highlighted the lack of support available for people living with cancer and other life limiting illnesses. Based on these needs, Murray Hall responded and secured funding to pilot a support service in Sandwell for people living with cancer at any stage of the illness including palliative and end of life care. The new service was based on a public health palliative care approach. The concept of a public health approach to palliative and end of life care was developed by Professor Allan Kellehear (1999), based on the World Health Organisation (WHO) models of health promotion and living well. The concept was extended to include living well to the end of life, and it was the first time health promotion was associated to the dying phase of life. Kellehear (1999) argued that by using a public health model in palliative care, it broadened and encompassed community involvement, reducing the isolation of dying people and increasing the capacity of the community to provide informal care and support (Kellehear, 2005).

The Murray Hall service partnership steering group was chaired by a local salaried GP, and included health, social care, and community members. A community member who had cared for her dying husband and had experienced a chasm between the medical professionals and themselves as patients and carers, choose the name "Bridges" for the new service. The service was launched in 2001 as a non-clinical palliative support service. Intrinsically the service had a public health community development approach, which encompassed the principles of health promotion and empowerment, supporting individuals to navigate systems, access information, and enabling them to be in control rather than passive receivers of care (Fawcett et al., 1993). It was unusual for a non-hospice community organisation to become the provider of the main community supportive palliative care service in Sandwell. The Bridges service model included:

- Care coordinators – to facilitate a Narrative Based Assessment, which involved listening to individuals tell their story and from their perspective identify their priority of needs, and supported them as appropriate.
- Information – ensured people had access to appropriate information to make informed choices and decisions.
- Navigation – supported people and carers to navigate health, social systems, housing, immigration systems etc.
- Advocacy – to speak and act on their behalf if required.
- Emotional support – ensured individuals had access to different forms of psychological support.
- Practical support – such as domestic support, respite, pop-in calls.
- Dedicated welfare rights officer – supported fast track benefit/finance support.
- Volunteer befrienders – provided informal companionship and support.
- Volunteer drivers – ensured people accessed vital appointments.
- Support group – enabled people to meet their peers and support each other.

Volunteers were an integral part of the service and were involved from the beginning providing support in different ways, mostly befriending and visiting people and their carers at home in the community. Volunteer drivers played a crucial role in supporting people to access essential treatment and medical appointments. It is not unusual for volunteers to be a feature of community development, and as part of a service they create powerful social bonds within the community, increasing awareness and support for those at end of life (Morris et al., 2012). The volunteers offered vital support, spending time with those who were lonely; they were formal volunteers offering informal befriending support. Traditionally end of life care volunteers within hospice settings in the UK were based within the hospice site (Morris et al., 2012), so it was unusual for the Bridges service volunteers to be out in the community visiting and supporting people in their own homes.

The Bridges care coordinators had a new non-traditional palliative care role that required flexibility. There is no one single definition of a care coordinator role but Yates (2004) found that the role of care coordinator was integral to the continuity of care as they were the one person who coordinated care across sectors and settings. Bridges care coordinators were navigator, advocate, organiser, assessor, advisor, befriender, and listener. In summary, they provided and enabled people to maintain their quality of life and remain at home. The care coordinators liaised and worked with other professionals from different disciplines, and attended different primary care multidisciplinary team meetings to provide integrated quality care.

While the Bridges service provided a non-clinical palliative care support to people in the community, Sandwell PCT secured National Lottery funding to establish a community clinical palliative care service called Hospice at Home (H@H) with specialist palliative care nurses. At the time, this model was different to other traditional hospice at home services that mainly included a team of health care assistants rather than specialist palliative care nurses. National directives incentivised an integrated approach (National Institute for Clinical Excellence, 2004; Walshe et al., 2007) which supported a holistic palliative care model of person-centred care. Murray Hall worked in collaboration with Sandwell PCT with a strategic decision to co-locate the new H@H team with the Bridges supportive care team at Murray Hall's main base within a new healthcare centre. Both services were steered in a direction that encouraged integration and cultural exchange. The PCT manager who established the H@H service importantly provided leadership and vision.

COOPERATION AND COLLABORATION

In 2004, the H@H service was launched, a community based specialist palliative care service for people with palliative and complex care needs. The team consisted of three specialist palliative care nurses and one administrator. At the same time, Murray Hall achieved sustainability of health funding and expanded the Bridges service across the borough to include all conditions. The team consisted of one manager, two care coordinators, and one administrator. Both the services were a hub and spoke model involving other organisations and services with the same aim to meet the needs of people at end of life and their families within the home setting. The main principle of the model was to provide integrated person-centred care to enable more people to have a realistic choice to achieve their preferred place of death. In most cases this was their home. A new partnership stakeholder group was established, with all partners signed up to the same shared goal of providing compassionate care and support and this ensured good communication and facilitated closer and effective working relationships. Grace et al. (2012) outline the features of a collaborative relationship, emphasising that collaboration is based on individuals being independent within a system signed up to the same goal.

The integrated approach ensured there was a seamless community palliative care provision for dying people and their families in Sandwell. The team members found that patients' confidence was enhanced in the knowledge that both teams were based together and able to discuss their care and provide coordinated support. The physical co-location of the two teams based together in one open-plan office was a key feature of the integrated approach. In a literature review of integrated working, Cameron et al. (2014) found that co-location was an important element in the success of joint working, as was building trust and respect between the professionals. This was evident within both teams as they complemented and supported each other with their different skills sets for a seamless service. The combined service design included multidisciplinary, multi-agency virtual integrated team working. This involved a stakeholder partnership approach of clinical and non-clinical organisations with a wider group of services and support, which included palliative care nurses, care coordinators, health care assistants, and bereavement support. They worked with the wider multidisciplinary teams, comprising district nurses, GPs, clinical nurse specialists, hospice day-care, physio- and occupational therapists, volunteers, other community organisations, social care housing, and local and national charities. Building good working relationships with all the different professionals was essential for effective quality care and support.

The service was underpinned by the national health priority to understand and support individuals' preference for place of care and death, which for the majority was home (Arnold et al., 2015). Both teams supported people with discussions about their preference for place of care and death. Within two years the two teams doubled their capacity to support more people in their preferred place and at the same time reduced unnecessary hospital admissions.

Case study 1: Supporting a young mother with children

Sarah (pseudonym) aged 43, married and mother of five children, was diagnosed with vulvar cancer with lung metastasis, she was referred by the DN to both Bridges and H@H services, and she was seen by the services within a few days. Each service team member coordinated either a joint visit or separate visits and updated each other following visits. The Bridges care coordinator found Sarah was physically struggling, especially when she picked up her youngest child as it caused her to have extensive bleeding and pain, which meant she did not leave the house but had not sought any medical help. The care coordinator contacted the hospital CNS who arranged for Sarah to attend the hospital and she received treatment several times a week, to manage her symptoms, and on the days she felt well enough she was able to leave the house again. A priority was to rapidly sort out the family finances and Bridges welfare rights officer visited Sarah secured extra benefits to reduce their finance anxieties and a Macmillan grant enabled Sarah to purchase a much needed new mattress.

The care coordinator identified that Sarah was struggling with daily living and arranged for domestic support to help her cope with daily tasks, such as family laundry, in particular the children's school uniforms. Also the impact of the diagnosis left Sarah feeling angry and frustrated, and agreed to see a counsellor. The H@H palliative care nurse spent time with Sarah discussing her concerns, anxieties about dying and support preparing the children for her death. The school nurse was made aware and offered to talk to the children, but, Sarah felt she needed to prepare the children herself.

Sarah chose to endure pain rather than take pain medication because of the side-effects. Family relationships were very strained, especially when all the children were at home as family outings were unaffordable. Both the services liaised to discuss the best course of support for Sarah and her family. A caravan holiday (Murray Hall asset) was offered, which they were delighted to accept and had a family holiday during the school half-term.

Her cancer had spread and Sarah needed urgent surgery, her main concern was childcare, during the day the older children were at school but no one to look after the youngest child. Her husband could not afford to take time off work or jeopardise losing his job. Several attempts were made by the care coordinator to contact the health visitor and social service but they were unresponsive. With surgery imminent the local Children Centre was contacted and the manager was empathetic, made an exception and offered the youngest a childcare place, which was a huge relief for Sarah. Her recovery coincided with the school summer holiday and so, Children Centre placement was secured for the youngest child for six weeks and the other children were allocated summer placement for three days, so Sarah could rest and recover from surgery during the summer. Sadly Sarah died before Christmas. It was only by working together that the best support was provided for Sarah, especially when compared to the difficulties encountered with outside agencies who were much more difficult to engage.

Case study 2: Dealing with shortcomings

Frank (pseudonym) aged 59 diagnosed with lung cancer two years earlier and suffered a breakdown at the time, recently had been informed he had extensive liver secondaries. He lived with his wife Mary (pseudonym) who had also been diagnosed with breast cancer recently and was awaiting news about treatment. Frank was referred to the Bridges service by the hospital clinical nurse specialist (CNS) for general support following the prognosis of extensive liver secondary.

On the day the care coordinator visited, Frank was unwell in bed after returning home from hospital. Mary was extremely upset about Frank's prognosis, they both struggled to come to terms that he would no longer have active treatment, and in particular how the news had been broken to them, they were told to go home and die. They had not had any follow up from their GP or CNS and they felt abandoned with little support or information. This came at a very emotional time for Mary unsure what treatment she needed for her own cancer diagnosis.

The care coordinator made Mary aware of the support available to them in the community, such as DN and H@H service, Mary felt reassured that the DNs would help with symptom control, but expressed that a referral to H@H at this stage was inappropriate as she felt her husband would "give up" if he was visited by a "hospice" service. The care coordinator contacted the CNS and informed her how Frank and Mary were feeling and their need for more information, and also referred Frank to the DN for a home visit. Unfortunately, the DN did not visit but instead referred directly to the H@H service, fortunately, with the Bridges and the H@H services based in the same office, they were able to advise them to hold back contacting the family until they were informed about the referral. The Bridges care coordinator contacted the DN case manager and was told that the DN and H@H palliative care nurse was visiting the family, which clearly was not the case. The co-location of the Bridges and the H@H service and the close working relationship prevented what could have been a very distressing situation and compromised patient care.

Frank was admitted to hospital again and was not expected to survive but his condition did improve slightly. Following the care coordinator's intervention the CNS spent some time with the family and discussed end of life care. It was at this point that a referral to H@H was made, this time with the family's blessing. The H@H palliative care nurse visited Frank at the hospital to assess for a care package and he returned home soon after with their input.

Trust with the family had been restored, they felt more supported, they were happy with the care and support they received. During this time Mary started radiotherapy treatment and the Bridges service supported Frank with respite care, and coordinated Mary's radiotherapy appointments with volunteer drivers to take her to hospital for several weeks of treatment. Frank died at home with his family present and Mary continued to be supported during her treatment and with her bereavement.

LEADERSHIP AND BLURRING OF BOUNDARIES

There were some key elements that contributed to the success of the interprofessional collaboration and integration. The first was the leadership of both the partner organisations aligned to the same vision and aims, which was communicated and shared with the teams. The team members were also committed to this vision and they liaised and worked as one team and supported each other with a good sense of camaraderie. The united leadership of both the organisations was very supportive of the teams working together as a seamless service, and a partnership approach was encouraged and supported at strategic level. This resonated with a key element in Cameron et al.'s (2014) study, that a strong management and leadership presence gives staff confidence and contributes to the success of collaboration.

The second important element was the co-location of the teams and the setting; both the teams were based at a health centre alongside Murray Hall's main office. The importance of this was that clinical team members were exposed to a third sector organisational culture of working alongside the community to empower them, which was very different to a clinical health environment. The charity managed a number of facilities within the health centre, such as a health information point, healthy café, and other community rooms. The centre also contained acute clinical services and a large GP practice. The partnership with the health centre was also innovative at the time and it meant that both clinical and non-clinical organisations were not just based in the community, but were working together *with* the community.

DISCUSSION: INTEGRATED TEAM WORKING

The location of the two teams together within Murray Hall's offices was significant, as it supported a hybrid culture where the boundaries of the two teams were blurred and together they offered individuals, carers, and their families a seamless, flexible, comprehensive, and compassionate palliative care service. The success of integrating the two teams was fully recognised by Sandwell PCT: as both the teams expanded they were relocated together to a larger office space to continue the integrated approach.

Enablers that promote integration

Leadership was pivotal to the success of the integrated approach of the clinical and non-clinical teams. Many of the enabling principles identified by Nancarrow et al. (2013) listed below in Table 6.1 were present as both teams worked collaboratively together for eight years.

There was a mutual respect for the prevailing culture of each umbrella organisation as they brought their expertise to the collaboration: PCT – healthcare and clinical governance, and Murray Hall – social model of health and community development. The combination of the two cultures contributed to the successful outcomes of supporting people at end of life. There was a shared understanding that a combination of a medical and social model provided effective supportive palliative end of life care. There was a close professional working relationship between the two teams and on many levels operated as one team for nearly a decade.

Barriers to integrating team working

One of the barriers to better integration was sharing electronic systems, not so much being connected to the interface of NHS systems, but the most challenging

TABLE 6.1 Principles of effective interdisciplinary teamwork

Ten principles that enable good interdisciplinary team work (Nancarrow et al., 2013)	
1. Leadership	6. Good communication
2. Shared values and vision	7. Appropriate mix of skills and staff
3. Culture of trust	8. Appropriate recruitment
4. Infrastructure and appropriate processes	9. Respect of roles and interdependence
5.Patient-focused care	10. Training and personal development

was information governance. After much effort and in anticipation, both teams were trained ready for rollout of a new shared IT system, however the momentum was lost when NHS national priorities changed. The structural changes within the NHS meant that the community health services were split from the commissioning element, and as the leadership and management changed, the H@H team were transferred to the local Hospital Trust and re-located. The two teams were no longer co-located and although they continued to work collaboratively, the same level of integration of support and care was not achieved after they were separated. Co-location was the most valuable and tangible advantage of the collaborative partnership – it enabled the smooth coordination and continuity of care and support for individuals. One particular patient expressed his confidence in knowing that both team members sat next to each other to arrange his care and support together. This was significant, as National Voices found that lack of integration was a real disadvantage for people as the following quote highlights: "The lack of joined-up care is the biggest frustration for patients, service users and carers" (National Voices, 2013, p. 1).

KEY POINTS

- In the last decade the NHS has undergone many structural changes and, in many cases, organisations face competing priorities and this has reduced their focus on third sector partnerships.
- Collaboration and integrated health and social care continue to be an ambition for patient-centred care, especially for patients with palliative care needs in the community.
- Our experience of an integrated approach is possible when the essential elements of leadership, shared values and vision, working towards the same goal, co-location, trust, and respect for all aspects of clinical and non-clinical care and flexibility are present.

REFERENCES

Abbott, S, Banks-Smith, J (2001) Can primary care groups and trust improve health. *BMJ*, 323, 89–92.

Arnold, E, Finucane, A, Oxenham, D (2015) Preferred place of death for patients referred to a specialist palliative care service. *BMJ Supportive & Palliative Care*, 5, 294–296. Available at: https://spcare.bmj.com/content/bmjspcare/5/3/294.full.pdf

Cameron, A, Lart, L, Bostock, L, Coomber, C (2014) Factors that promote and hinder joint and integrated working between health and social care: a review of research literature. *Health and Social Care in the Community*, 22(3), 225–233.

Department for Communities and Local Government (2011) *English indices of deprivation 2010*. DCLG, London.

Department of Health (2000) *NHS Plan*. HMSO, London.

Fawcett, S, Paine, A, Francico, V, Vliet, M (1993) Promoting health through community development. In Glenwick, D, Jason, L (eds) *Promoting health and mental health in children, youth, and families*. Springer Publishing Company, New York.

Grace, M, Coventry, L, Batterham, D (2012) The role of interagency collaboration in "joined-up" case management. *Journal of Interprofessional Care*, 26, 141–149.

Kellehear, A (1999) *Health promoting palliative care*. University Press, Melbourne.

Kellehear, A (2005) *Compassionate cities*. Routledge, Oxford.

Lloyd, L, Wait, S (2005) *Integrated care – a guide for policymakers*. Alliance for Health and the Future, London.

Morris, S, Wilmot, A, Hill, M, Ockenden, N, Payne, S (2012) A narrative literature review of the contribution of volunteers in end of life care services. *Palliative Medicine*, 27(5), 428–436.

Nancarrow, S, Booth, A, Ariss, S, Smith, T, Enderby, P, Roots, A (2013) Ten principles of good interdisciplinary team work. *Human Resources for Health*, 11(19). Available at: http://www.human-resources-health.com/11/1/19

National Institute for Clinical Excellence (2004) *Guidance on cancer services. Improving supportive and palliative care for adults with cancer*. The Manual. NICE, London.

National Voices (2013) *Principles for integrated care*. National Voices, London. Available at: https://www.nationalvoices.org.uk/publications/our-publications/principles-integrated-care

Walshe, C, Chew-Graham, C, Todd, C (2007) Evaluating partnerships working: lessons for palliative care. *European Journal of Cancer Care*, 16, 48–54.

Wilson, M, Meldrum, M (2013) A history of hospice and palliative medicine. In Lutz, S, Chow, E, and Hoskins, P (eds) *Radiation oncology in palliative cancer care*. Wiley-Blackwell, London.

Yates, P (2004) Cancer care coordinators: realising the potential for improving the patient journey. *Cancer Forum*, 28(3), 129–132.

CHAPTER 7

Psychological care

Everybody's business?

....

Dave Roberts

OUTLINE

Palliative care has a well-established holistic approach, and an emphasis on emotional and psychosocial care. This holistic approach has led to an assumption within palliative care that the psychological or psychosocial aspects of care are a fundamental and unifying feature underlying the work of the whole team. However, as O'Connor & Fisher (2011) point out, roles are not always well defined, teamwork does not take place automatically, and the psychosocial aspects of care may actually be the most contested. This is well summed up in their quote "...everybody thinks that everybody can do it and they can't" (p. 194). This chapter is an exploration of what we mean by psychological care, who does it, and how it is carried out.

BACKGROUND: DIFFERENT TERMINOLOGY AND ROLES

Whereas all members of the palliative care team members may feel a personal investment in psychological aspects of care, some members of the team will have specific skills, training, or responsibilities. They may also use terminology in ways that are meaningful within their own professional group, and draw on specific concepts from counselling, psychology, and psychotherapies. Meanings can be complex and nuanced and benefit from clarification. The following are definitions of some key terminology in this area which may be helpful.

Psychological – the emotional and cognitive aspects of the patient's experience and care, including assessment and interventions.
Psychosocial – this includes the emotional aspects of care but within an explicit social context.

DOI: 10.4324/9781351113472-7

Social – may include emotional but also embraces family and organisational dynamics, and may include finances, and the legal context of families.

O'Connor & Fisher (2011) argue that both doctors and nurses in palliative care may claim expertise in all aspects of the care of the dying patient, social workers would have a claim to particular expertise in the psychosocial, and psychologists argue for a particular role in psychological assessment and interventions. Other groups, including chaplains and occupational therapists, have a claim to provide important aspects of psychosocial care. This can result in competition or a struggle to differentiate roles and identify their place in the team.

Given this diversity of roles, and potential for tension between them, it is important that all professional groups in palliative care work together for the benefit of the patient, by sharing common aims. However, more than this is needed. To avoid role conflict, professionals need to develop self-awareness and mutual support systems. This will often include joint interprofessional training and education programmes, but also policies and structures that nurture interprofessional teamworking (O'Connor & Fisher 2011).

LEVELS OF PSYCHOLOGICAL CARE

One significant attempt to reconcile these tensions within the field of cancer and palliative care was undertaken by the National Institute for Health and Care Excellence (then known as National Institute for Clinical Excellence). "Improving Supportive and Palliative Care for Adults with Cancer" (NICE 2004) provided guidance and defined service models on a range of supportive and palliative care activities. Underlying principles included the importance of interprofessional communication and coordination of care and the value of partnerships between patients and carers and health and social care professionals to achieve best outcomes. This included multi-agency and multidisciplinary team working.

Importantly, it established four levels of psychological care, identifying the roles of different groups of staff in psychological assessment and intervention. It should be noted that self-help and informal support run alongside all of the four levels.

Psychological support level 1: All health and social care professionals

Assessments by professionals at level 1, the baseline for all health and social care, should recognise psychological distress, avoid causing psychological harm, and be aware of the limits of competence, and when to refer on for specialist assessment. Interventions at this level include honest and compassionate communication, treating patients and carers with kindness, dignity, and respect, establishing and maintaining supportive relationships, and providing information about the emotional and support services available to them. Relationships and communication are central to all of palliative care practice.

Psychological support level 2: Professionals with additional expertise

At level 2, professionals should be trained to screen for psychological distress at key points in the patient pathway. This screening should include the impact of their condition on their lives, mood, family relationships, and work. The aim of screening should be to elicit worries and concerns, and the process itself may lead to a resolution. If not, they may be referred for specialist support.

Level 2 involves psychological techniques such as problem-solving delivered by trained and supervised health and social care professionals. This level has been associated with specialist nurses, among others, following specialist training, and there are good examples of nurses being trained to effectively deliver problem-solving, with impressive outcomes in terms of patient coping and improved mood (Sharpe et al., 2004; Strong et al., 2008).

Psychological support level 3: Trained and accredited professionals

Assessment at this level concerns differentiating between moderate and severe levels of psychological need and being able to refer on to mental health specialists. In terms of interventions, it is specified at this level that trained, accredited, and supervised practitioners deliver therapies such as anxiety management or solution-focused therapy according to an explicit theoretical framework. It aims to manage mild to moderate levels of psychological distress including anxiety, depression and anger, personal relationships, and spiritual issues.

Psychological support level 4: Mental health specialists

Level 4 is where mental health specialists (including psychiatrists, psychologists, mental health nurses, for example) provide assessment and diagnosis of more complex and severe psychological problems. Their interventions target moderate to severe mental health problems, including depression and anxiety, organic brain syndromes, drug-related problems, personality disorder, and psychotic illness.

The guidance also has separate sections on social support and spiritual support services, areas where there is overlap with psychological support. There is an acknowledgement of some of the problems providing psychological services: limited availability of specialist professionals, a lack of agreement on what needs to be provided across different professional groups, and a lack of coordination resulting in limited access to specialist resources.

Whilst this service model established a unifying framework for psychological care, the implementation of the model was left to local service providers and commissioners, and there is room for interpretation, for example, about the level of training needed to raise professionals from level 1 to levels 2 and 3. There are also ambiguities and overlap between different levels. It has also become clear that, as education programmes have evolved in response to the guidance, training alone may not be enough to develop the necessary skills, and that ongoing supervision and support are necessary for the maintenance of skills in the longer term (Mannix et al., 2006).

This chapter will now go on to discuss the range of psychological problems encountered in palliative care practice. These are framed around the four levels of assessment and intervention for the purpose of illustration, though in practice different conditions do fit neatly within these levels.

LEVEL 1: HUMAN SUFFERING AND DISTRESS

Psychological problems in palliative care have often been characterised as a form of suffering, an experience of severe distress, encompassing physical, psychological, social, and spiritual dimensions of being. It arises out of a sense that the integrity of the person, or their continued existence, is threatened (Cassel, 1982). This represents the existential crisis of facing our own mortality and death, arguable the most serious challenge that we as humans face in the course of our lives (Yalom, 2008).

Central to suffering are threats to our sense of self or personhood, personal and bodily integrity, and personal identity, the elements that identify us as a person. Threats can take many forms. Loss of independence or dignity, loss of control, physical functions and capacity, and loss of occupational and family role all contribute to a sense of suffering. In addition, the meaning attached to these losses and associated events like pain or other symptoms, contribute. Pain may be bearable as a short-term unpleasant experience, but if it signifies impending loss of dignity or death, it may become an overwhelming and unbearable experience.

The concept of psychological distress describes a continuum of feelings including vulnerability, sadness, anxiety, and depression. Distress may be experienced by an individual or by couples or other family units, and this may be transient, or long lasting and disabling (Carolan et al., 2015). Although common, it may only be clinically significant and require treatment in about one third of all cases (Howell & Olsen, 2011).

Personal distress can be recognised by people's observed behaviour and by what they say, and how they say it. Active engagement and interaction with the patient and family gives opportunities to observe both behaviour and communication. Responses to distress include the most fundamental and important human interventions: being with the person, doing things with and for them in a compassionate and caring way, forming, maintaining and ending relationships. Empathic responses, that demonstrate understanding of the other person's feelings, are central to responding to distress. All health professionals should have the capacity to respond to distress in a compassionate and empathic manner, and case study 1 illustrates how this is often weaved into the fabric of care.

Case study 1: Recognising and responding to distress

Sheila is a district nurse and visits Mr Whitehouse for the first time. He has just been discharged from hospital where he was having treatment for metastatic cancer of the colon. Mr Whitehouse, who is 72, knows his expectation of life is short, and he wants to die at home. He is supported by his wife and two adult children also live nearby. Sheila will be working with the family with the support of a community palliative care nurse.

Sheila understands from experience the importance of a first meeting as an opportunity to get to know each other and for working together. On entering the house, she is greeted by Mrs Whitehouse, who she notices looks worried. She shows Sheila into the living room, and introduces her husband, then leaves them. Meeting Mr Whitehouse, Sheila consciously engages in eye contact with him, and notices that, after briefly returning her gaze, he looks away. Sitting on the next chair to him, she asks about his recent stay in hospital, and how he is feeling. Whilst responding, Sheila observes that he looks distracted and preoccupied.

After some discussion of his recent hospital admission and his understanding of his current condition, Sheila asks Mr Whitehouse "Is there something that you are concerned about?" He breaks into tears, and says he knows he is going to die, and he accepts that, but he fears being a burden on his wife, and he worries that she will not be able to cope. Sheila shows empathy by reflecting back to him some of the more significant things that he has said "you are worried about being a burden ... that Mrs Whitehouse won't be able to cope..." She instinctively reaches out to briefly hold his hand, and he smiles in return. Sheila suggests that his wife joins them, and together they discuss what support will be available to his wife, and how they can record his wishes for his future care.

LEVEL 2: PERSONAL REACTIONS AND COPING

The concepts of suffering and distress have value in understanding the person as a whole. However, in practice, it is often useful to identify more specific personal reactions. These are often a presenting problem, and should be picked up by Holistic Needs Assessment (Macmillan, n.d.). They provide a focus for interventions. They may include:

- Anger.
- Denial.
- Anxiety, including panic.
- Rumination and bleak thoughts.
- Poor concentration and confusion.
- Withdrawal and social isolation.
- Low mood, depression.
- Demoralisation.

These are determined by many factors, including personality, and they can be understood as representing the person's coping response to the situation. Coping is an attempt to deal with a situation that taxes the person's emotional resources. Coping behaviours can be characterised as:

- Problem-focused coping (efforts to manage the problem).
- Emotion-focused coping (efforts taken to regulate distress).
- Meaning-based coping (efforts to maintain well-being).

(Folkman & Greer, 2000)

Effective coping means that the person ends up feeling more in control. For this reason problem-focused coping is usually seen as more effective than emotion-focused coping, e.g. distraction from rather than focusing on the problem, which may make the person feel better in the short term without resolving the underlying problem. Meaning-based coping is more likely to result in a better long-term outcome as it promotes well-being, reflection, and finding meaning in the experience. Problem-solving treatment aims to support effective coping by making problems more manageable (Areán, 2009), and an example of its use is given in case study 2.

Another way of understanding personal reactions is in terms of personal resilience. That is, the person's ability to react in a positive way in the face of significant threat or adversity. Factors that promote resilience include: self-esteem, self-efficacy, flexibility, humour, and a capacity for regulating emotions (Agaibi & Wilson, 2005).

In addition to these personal reactions, there may be factors in the situation or the interaction between the situation and the person, which determine the reaction. Trauma as a result of difficult experiences is associated with intrusive thoughts or images, distressing dreams, and anxiety. These may be brief and transient or long-term, persistent, and disabling, a condition termed posttraumatic stress disorder (PTSD). This range of reactions can occur in palliative care settings, associated with unsettling experiences, bad news or, for example, periods spent in the intensive care unit. It is important to be aware that not all traumatic experiences lead to a traumatic reaction. Posttraumatic growth can occur where the person reappraises their life and personal priorities, finds new meaning in life, enhanced relationships, and spirituality (Connerty & Knott, 2013).

Case study 2: Coping and problem solving

Tony, a 54 year old man, has been diagnosed with oesophageal cancer. He is finding it hard to come to terms with his poor prognosis. He feels it is unfair to be facing death at such a young age. He is also very angry that he has worked hard to set up and run his own business for many years and now will not achieve his aim of retiring early and enjoying the fruits of his labours. He is feeling very stuck, in that he cannot talk about any future plans or wishes, as this reminds him of the unfairness of the situation, but he wants to make the most of his time left.

Helen is Tony's palliative care nurse and she is trying to support him through this period of adjustment. Helen admits to colleagues that she finds his anger difficult, as he can come across as resentful and uncooperative. She finds it impossible to directly address his anger with him as he responds to this aggressively. She has spent time listening to him but he seems unable to get beyond his anger and resentment.

Helen has supervision from a psychologist and they discuss alternative approaches. They agree to try problem-solving, with supervision from the psychologist. This is a structured approach that requires the therapist to work with the patient to first find the motivation to change, then identify the problem or problems, brainstorm potential solutions, then identify the most practical options and plan steps to implement them, then review.

In the first session, Tony is helped by Helen to recognise how much frustration both he and his family are experiencing. They identify that previously he was very active, walking and cycling, and this helped him cope with work pressures. The problem is identified as Tony no longer using this as a coping strategy, and they agree he could try to reintroduce walking in the countryside with his wife. A plan is made and reviewing his progress helps Tony to talk about his feelings without them being directly confronted. He is angry that he cannot walk as far as he did before but he is able to take satisfaction from walking again and enjoying the countryside. This is how he had planned to spend his retirement and he now has some time to enjoy and share it with his wife. Discussions between Helen and Tony become more open as a result and they are able to move on to other aspects of Tony's future care and treatment.

LEVEL 3: ANXIETY

Anxiety and worry are a normal part of life, associated with uncertainty and a sense of apprehension. Anxiety in everyday life is a response to the perception of threat. If the response results in successful coping, then the threat is resolved and the anxiety dissipates. In most cases, anxiety and worry may be uncomfortable but not distressing. However, if the sense of threat is not resolved, then it may become severe, long-lasting, or prevent us from leading our lives. Within the palliative care context, there are numerous potential triggers for anxiety. These include bad news or changes in health status, hospital appointments and waiting for test results, and unpleasant procedures. The extent to which a person will feel anxious depends on a number of factors. These include the individual tendency to be anxious (trait anxiety), the nature or unpredictability of the situation, and the meaning that the person ascribes to that situation. We should always be cautious about identifying the anxiety with the patient's personality (the "anxious patient"), however, as the experience of anxiety is always about the individual perception of threat.

Anxiety can manifest in many ways, and affects the whole person. Physical effects of anxiety are very prominent, and can include rapid pulse (tachycardia) and rapid shallow breathing (hyperventilation). Understandably, people who are feeling anxious and who experience these symptoms may interpret them as signs of a cata-strophic illness event like cardiac arrest. Also, long term health conditions such as cancer are often associated with a raised awareness (hypervigilance) about physical symptoms and what they represent; does a new pain signify a recurrence of cancer? Anxiety and pain are linked: pain makes people feel anxious and the experience of pain is heightened by anxiety.

Psychologically, anxiety is associated with fearfulness, apprehension, and uncer-tainty, poor concentration, worrying thoughts, and sometimes a sense of impending doom. Behaviour also shows signs of anxiety: agitation and restlessness. Anxiety may have a profound effect on the patient's ability to absorb and retain information and cooperate with professional staff in the process of decision-making. Any actions that provide comfort, given by family and other carers, may help the patient to cope with anxiety, and also actions that promote a sense of personal control, i.e. manag-ing the uncertainty.

There is a range of therapeutic interventions that help the person dealing with anxiety. Relaxation may be promoted by relaxation training, which usually involves progressive muscle relaxation, combined with deep breathing exercises and guided imagery (Pollak et al., 2015). Relaxation can also be induced using music therapy, which is well established in many palliative care centres (Warth et al., 2014). Anxiety management includes specific techniques to enable the patient to cope more effec-tively. These include distraction, finding a focus outside of the self that takes atten-tion away from anxious preoccupations, and challenging anxious thoughts.

Anxiety management is also practised within the framework of cognitive behav-iour therapy (CBT), which uses models for understanding how anxiety develops and is maintained. Actions can then be taken to stop these anxious processes (Kennerley et al., 2016). For example, the cognitive model of panic attacks, severe episodes of acute anxiety, shows that attacks are usually triggered by an anxious thought. Identifying this trigger enables the patient to recognise when an attack may occur and thereby prevent it. Similarly, health anxiety (sometimes with hypervigilance) can lead to a morbid preoccupation with physical symptoms. This can be helped by dis-tracting the patient from the physical sensations, and challenging the more negative explanations for these, as in case study 3.

Case study 3: Anxiety and anxiety management

Janet is 45 and has a diagnosis of ovarian cancer. She was diagnosed over a year ago and had not expected to live so long. She made preparations for dying, including discus-sions with her children and making "memory boxes" for them. However, she is currently disease-free and struggling to deal with the uncertainty of her circumstances.

Janet attends the local hospice day care once a week, whilst her husband is at work and her children at school. She values the company and the emotional support. However, she is troubled by anxiety, particularly about her health. She interprets any new sensation, any aches or pains, as signs of disease recurrence, and this triggers rumination about her illness and her future. She describes "dark thoughts" that get worse when she is alone.

The team in the hospice discuss Janet's care with her and agree a plan to support her. She is offered attendance at relaxation sessions run by the occupational therapist and sessions with the music therapist, which she accepts. The hospice doctor has had training in CBT-based anxiety management and makes appointments with Janet to discuss how this could help. Janet and Dr Jones make a list of things that could cause her realistic concern and should lead to discussion with the oncology team. They then agree that Janet should distract herself from any anxious thoughts that do not relate to these features. They agree ways she could do this, including thinking positive thoughts about her children and listening to music (helped by the music therapist). She could also challenge these thoughts and replace them with more positive ones, e.g. "this is just a twinge, everyone gets them, and it does not mean my disease has come back". With support, Janet becomes less anxious and, although she still has occasional anxious and dark thoughts, she is more able to manage them and keep them in perspective.

LEVEL 4: DEPRESSION

Depression presents particular challenges for the interprofessional team. This is because it can be understood in a variety of different ways. Depression is a state of low mood. As an emotional state it could be seen as ubiquitous in the palliative care setting, a natural reaction to a grim situation, or a stage of grief in response to actual and impending loss. It may be part of a spiritual or existential state, of loss of meaning or purpose towards the end of life. This could be allied to pain, or a component of total pain. As an emotional state, it can be placed at one end of a continuum of sadness, i.e. transient sadness in reaction to the situation, more prolonged sadness in bereavement, and the persistent unvarying mood which characterises depression. Viewed from this perspective, the *spectral model of depression*, it may be interpreted as a natural condition that may require compassionate support, but should not be pathologised or medicalised, i.e. treated as an illness (Ng et al., 2015).

However, depression can also be seen as an illness, one that has clear, diagnosable features, and one that responds to specific treatments and has different qualities from sadness (Rayner et al., 2010). On the one hand, patients, family, and professionals may wish to avoid the stigma of mental illness associated with depression, on the other, patients may feel a sense of relief if their emotional state is recognised and treated. Different health professionals may view depression as an emotional state, a symptom, or an illness (Ng et al., 2015) and see themselves having a primary role in its management in palliative care, for example, the social worker in a complex family situation, the chaplain in a patient with spiritual distress, or the doctor in prescribing antidepressants.

One challenge, therefore, is to make an assessment that allows the distinction between sadness and depression to be made. Another problem is in the diagnosis of depression, as some features of depression can also be caused by the patient's illness or treatment: in a physically healthy person, sleep and appetite disturbance are reliable diagnostic criteria. However, these cannot be relied on for diagnosis in the physically ill.

Managing depression in palliative care

Because of the ambiguity in the ways we understand depression, it is important to base its management on sound interprofessional assessment. The first stage of this is screening for depression, if it is suspected that a patient is depressed on the basis of their presentation and behaviour. This can be achieved using either a structured interview or questionnaire. The most basic interview involves asking specific questions that have been shown to identify key features of depression. This is simply asking the single question "Are you depressed?" or the two questions:

"During the last month, have you been bothered by feeling down, depressed, or hopeless?"
"During the last month, have you been bothered by having little interest or pleasure in doing things?"

These questions address fundamental characteristics of depression: persistent, unvarying low mood and loss of interest in things (anhedonia), neither of which would be caused by physical illness alone (Chochinov et al., 1997). A more comprehensive assessment, based on non-physical symptoms, is posed by the Hospital Anxiety and Depression Scale (HADS). This has seven questions relating to depressed mood and seven relating to anxiety, with a score range of between 0–21, with 11–21 being clinically significant (Zigmond & Snaith., 1983). An alternative screening tool for non-verbal patients is the Distress Thermometer, which only requires the patient to point to where they are feeling on a visual analogue scale (Roth et al., 1998). These assessments can be used for both anxiety and depression, which are often found together. Treatments for depression include antidepressant therapy, cognitive behaviour therapy, shown in case study 4, and mindfulness which has been proven to be effective in preventing relapse of depression (Kennerley et al., 2016).

Case 4: Depression or demoralisation?

Lillian is 35 year old teacher with a small child, has breast cancer with a poor prognosis, though currently free of any symptoms. On attending the oncology outpatients clinic, she reports tiredness, being unable to work, doing less at home, and avoiding friends. The staff in outpatients are concerned about her but divided about what to do. Some of the outpatient nurses feel her mood is understandable and that it would help if her family and friends tried to get her out more. Her breast cancer specialist nurse, however, thinks she may be depressed and would like to get professional support for her. She asks Lillian to fill in the HADS, and she scores 14 on the Depression scale, 9 on the Anxiety scale. On the basis of this screening assessment, which suggests a clinical case of depression, and borderline score on anxiety, Lilian is referred to the psycho-oncology clinic at the hospital.

Dan, the mental health specialist nurse in the psycho-oncology clinic, is trained in cognitive behaviour therapy (CBT). He assesses Lillian and decides on a therapy designed to help depression, *activity scheduling*. When people are depressed, they lose the motivation to do things, and they no longer enjoy their life. According to the cognitive model of depression, doing less feeds into a sense of hopelessness, with no sense of achievement or pleasure. The aim of activity scheduling therapy is to re-establish activities and record the sense of achievement and pleasure that results. The record is then discussed in outpatient sessions with the therapist, where progress is reviewed. Activity can then be scaled up, becoming increasingly rewarding and pleasurable. Mood is also assessed regularly, so that improvements can recognised and celebrated.

Lillian makes good progress over the coming weeks, increasing her range of activities, getting out more, and reversing her social withdrawal by meeting more friends outside the home. Whilst Lillian did die from breast cancer, her final months were rewarding for her and spent in the company of family and friends.

THE DEMANDS OF PSYCHOLOGICAL CARE

Relationships, with patients and their carers, and with colleagues, can be the most satisfying and rewarding, but also the most demanding aspects of work in palliative care. Investing ourselves in our work, and managing our emotions to ensure our patients or clients feel secure and cared for, requires emotional labour (Smith, 2012). Other causes of stress include workload and inadequate resources, role conflict, and constant exposure to the distress and suffering of others (Peters et al., 2012). This takes its toll, and in the long term, the negative side effects of emotional labour can be described as burnout, vicarious trauma, or compassion fatigue. These may lead to exhaustion, demoralisation, loss of job satisfaction, or depression.

However, there are things that we can do to protect ourselves, and turn our experience of the trauma of others into posttraumatic growth for ourselves. Factors that can promote resilience in the face of adversity include building positive nurturing relationships, seeing positive benefits in adversity, developing emotional insight and becoming more reflective (Jackson et al., 2007). It is also helpful to recognise that compassion can bring both satisfaction and fatigue, and the Compassion Fatigue Awareness Project has developed a self-scoring device for assessing these, and this can be used as a point of personal reflection (access here: https://proqol.org/uploads /ProQOL_5_English_Self-Score.pdf).

However, the working environment also has a role. Supportive management can promote self-care within the workplace, through mentorship and supervisory relationships, and meetings to reflect and debrief after traumatic incidents (Peters et al,. 2012). Role conflict is itself very stressful, so actions taken to resolve this will lead to a more harmonious and less stressful working environment. Education and ongoing professional development are also supportive, and if this is done within the frame of interprofessional education, it will provide opportunities for both formal and informal support with the emotional demands of palliative care (Shaw et al., 2016).

KEY POINTS

- Psychological aspects of care are an essential part of the holistic approach of the palliative care team, and each team member may have a particular contribution to make.
- However, some team members will have specialist expertise in psychological assessment and treatment.
- The NICE four level model enables distinctions to be made between assessments and interventions undertaken by different members of the team, based on their skills and training.
- Psychological care is one of the most demanding aspects of palliative care, and individuals, teams, and organisations need to develop supportive strategies and structures to manage this.

ADDITIONAL RESOURCES

Compassion Fatigue Awareness Project: http://www.compassionfatigue.org/index.html
NHS Mindfulness: https://www.nhs.uk/conditions/stress-anxiety-depression/mindfulness/

REFERENCES

Agaibi, CE, Wilson, JP (2005) Trauma, PTSD, and resilience. *Trauma, Violence, & Abuse*, 6(3), 195–216.

Areán, PA (2009) Problem-solving therapy. *Psychiatric Annals*, 39(9), 854–858, 860–862.

Carolan, CM, Smith, A, Forbat, L (2015) Conceptualising psychological distress in families in palliative care: findings from a systematic review. *Palliative Medicine*, 29(7), 605–632. doi: 10.1177/0269216315575680

Cassel, EJ (1982) The nature of suffering and the goals of medicine. *The New England Journal of Medicine*, 306(11), 639–645.

Chochinov, HM, Wilson, KG, Enns, M, Lander, S (1997) "Are you depressed?" Screening for depression in the terminally ill. *American Journal of Psychiatry*, 154, 674–676.

Connerty, TJ, Knott, V (2013) Promoting positive change in the face of adversity: experiences of cancer and post-traumatic growth. *European Journal of Cancer Care*, 22, 334–344.

Folkman, S, Greer, S (2000) Promoting psychological well-being in the face of serious illness: when theory, research and practice inform each other. *Psycho-oncology*, 9, 11–19.

Howell, D, Olsen, K (2011) Distress-the 6th vital sign. *Current Oncology*, 18(5), 208–210.

Jackson, D, Firtko, A, Edenborough, M (2007) Personal resilience as a strategy for surviving and thriving in the face of workplace adversity: a literature review. *Journal of Advanced Nursing*, 60(1), 1–9.

Kennerley, H, Kirk, J, Westbrook, D (2016) *An introduction to cognitive behaviour therapy. Skills & applications* (3rd ed.). SAGE, London.

Macmillan (n.d.) Holistic needs assessments. Accessed at: https://www.macmillan.org.uk/healthcare-professionals/innovation-in-cancer-care/holistic-needs-assessment

Mannix, KA, Blackburn, IM, Garland, A, Gracie, J, Moorey, S, Reid, B, Scott, J (2006) Effectiveness of brief training in cognitive behaviour therapy techniques for palliative care practitioners. *Palliative Medicine*, 20, 579–584.

National Institute for Health and Clinical Excellence (2004) *Improving supportive and palliative care for adults with cancer.* NICE, London.

Ng, F, Crawford, G, Chur-Hansen, A (2015) Depression means different things: a qualitative study of psychiatrists' conceptualization of depression in the palliative care setting. *Palliative and Supportive Care*, 13(5), 1223–1230. doi: 10.1017/S1478951514001187

O'Connor M, Fischer, C (2011) Exploring the dynamics of interdisciplinary palliative care teams in providing psychosocial care: "Everybody thinks everybody can do it, and they can't." *Journal of Palliative Medicine*, 14(2), 191–196.

Peters, L, Cant, R, Sellick, K, O'Connor, M, Lee, S, Burney, S (2012) Is work stress in palliative care nurses a cause for concern? A literature review. *International Journal of Palliative Nursing*, 18(11), 561–567.

Pollak, K, Lyna, P, Bilheimer, A, et al. (2015) A brief relaxation intervention for pain delivered by palliative care physicians: a pilot study. *Palliative Medicine*, 29, 569–70.

Rayner, L, Higginson, IJ, Price, A, Hotopf, M (2010) *The management of depression in palliative care: European clinical guidelines.* Department of Palliative Care, Policy & Rehabilitation, London (www.kcl.ac.uk/schools/medicine/depts/palliative)/European Palliative Care Research Collaborative (www.epcrc.org).

Roth, AJ, Kornblith, AB, Batel-Copel, L, Peabody, E, Scher, HI, Holland, JC (1998) Rapid screening for psychologic distress in men with prostate carcinoma: a pilot study. *Cancer*, 82, 1904–1908.

Sharpe, M, Strong, V, Allen, K, Rush, R, Maguire, P, House, A, Ramirez, AC (2004) Management of major depression in outpatients attending a cancer centre: a preliminary evaluation of a multicomponent cancer nurse-delivered intervention. *British Journal of Cancer*, 90, 310–313.

Shaw, J, Kearney, C, Glenns, B, McKay, S (2016) Interprofessional team building in the palliative home care setting: use of a conceptual framework to inform a pilot evaluation. *Journal of Interprofessional Care*, 30(2), 262–264.

Smith, P (2012) *The emotional labour of nursing revisited: can nurses still care?* 2nd ed. Palgrave Macmillan, Basingstoke.

Strong, V, Waters, R, Hibberd, C, Murray, G, Wall, L, Walker, J, McHugh, G, Walker, A, Sharpe, M (2008) Management of depression for people with cancer (SMaRT oncology 1): a randomised trial. *The Lancet*, 372, 40–48.

Warth, M, Kessler, J, Koenig, J, Wormit, AF, Hillecke, TK, Bardenheuer, HJ (2014) Music therapy to promote psychological and physiological relaxation in palliative care patients: protocol of a randomized controlled trial. *BMC Palliative Care*, 13, 1–7.

Yalom, ID (2008) Staring at the sun: overcoming the terror of death. *The Humanistic Psychologist*, 36(3–4), 283–297. doi: 10.1080/08873260802350006

Zigmond, AS, Snaith, RP (1983) The hospital anxiety and depression scale. *Acta Psychiatrica Scandinavica*, 67, 361–370.

CHAPTER 8

Compassionate communities

Working with marginalised populations

....

Aliki Karapliagkou

OUTLINE

Palliative care relies upon interprofessional collaborations to meet its holistic objectives. Palliative care specialists, other clinical practitioners, medical technologists, palliative care nurses, counsellors, and chaplaincy services commonly collaborate to address end of life care needs. A less conspicuous partner is the community, consisting of the immediate and extended family, as well as neighbours and members of the same locality. Citizen led initiatives such as the Compassionate Communities (Wegleitner et al., 2016), as well as primary care led community development programmes (Abel et al., 2018), engage professionals and citizens in end of life interactions. They recognise that dying, grief, and caregiving take place at home and in the community, where sickness and health, birth and death, and love and loss coexist and are experienced in proximity to one another.

The present chapter will consider how the transfer and application of interprofessional collaborations in community settings may promote social inclusion among marginalised ethnic minority communities. Compassionate Cities, as local authority led public health interventions, employ professional-community partnerships to facilitate social integration. The aim is to deliver health-promoting outcomes among people with end of life care needs as well as all citizens. Consideration of the lived experience of racialisation affecting African-Caribbean communities in the UK will help us understand how we may be able to form partnerships that include grassroots end of life care organisation. The objective is to identify how we may more effectively represent and most importantly work through structures that are meaningful and serve transformational purposes for socially disadvantaged groups.

From a historical perspective, palliative care has varied considerably, referring to experiences and practices that are far from homogeneous. As a primarily community matter, the practice of care for the end of life in pre-industrial societies

DOI: 10.4324/9781351113472-8

was ritualistically performed to assert cultural values and negotiate social status. In modern times, the care of terminally ill people became synonymous with the application of medical treatments, curative knowledge, and technological innovations in hospitals and other institutional settings. However, historical analyses by McManners (1981) and Aries (1974) indicate that despite pressures to comply with trends set by a progressively medicalised culture, care for the dying and bereaved remained dependent upon socio-economic conditions. Poverty and social disadvantage encouraged adaptive cultural creativity in responses to loss.

The modern palliative care movement and public health end of life care initiatives revisit and reinvent the principles of community care that helped populations deal with death and dying in past times. Citizens are employed in supportive and voluntary roles in institutional and community settings to deliver personalised care, provide social support, and relieve social isolation. Public health end of life care responds to evidence that social exclusion is linked to worse health outcomes and mortality (Holt-Lunstad and Smith, 2012), and Compassionate Cities (Kellehear, 2005; 1999) advocate that health does not equate with the absence of disease. Therefore, wellbeing should be pursued at all stages of life, including the end of life. This can be achieved through the social incorporation of the frail and elderly, people with life-limiting conditions, the bereaved, caregivers, and people at increased risk of morbidity and mortality into social life.

Compassionate Cities as a public health policy framework lead a societal reorientation towards the end of life and its care, while local authorities and citizens are invested in its definition and practice. Implementation is driven by the Compassionate Cities Charter (Kellehear, 2016), consisting of 13 actions that prescribe initiatives and adaptations in social institutions, services, community, cultural and voluntary organisations, as well as environmental interventions that incorporate end of life care into daily life. Compassion as an ethical imperative towards the end of life becomes integrated into local authority health policy.

The main challenge in the process of adoption and implementation of the Compassionate Cities Charter has been its reliance upon naturalistic care networks. This may be ethically desirable but difficult to evidence with reference to objective deliverables beneficial to health systems (Collins et al., 2020). As this chapter will illustrate, marginalised communities independently construct care networks and enhance the end of life with meaning based upon their unique social circumstances and historical experiences. Taking these care relationships into account, will serve to sharpen our observational and interpretative skills to perceive insights that lie beyond the obvious and narrow sense of our assumptive world and respond to them sensitively in interprofessional palliative care practices. Constructive conceptualisation of naturalistic community care directly acknowledges its contribution to health systems, but also appreciates their role in restoring trust and cohesion. Social capital counteracts the compromising effects of inequalities upon health and wellbeing and promotes quality of life for all in modern societies (Marmot, 2015).

BACKGROUND: COMMUNITY ENGAGEMENT IN END OF LIFE CARE

Involving family members in the care of people with life-limiting conditions was the first step taken to open up palliative care (Glajchen, 2004; Waldro et al., 2005; Hebert and Schulz, 2006). Much research has been dedicated to the study of caregiver burden to enable their involvement in care and understand the kind of support from which they stand to benefit (Costa-Requena et al., 2015; Fried et al., 2004). People at the end of life need increased care delivered at home and in the community (Hudson and Payne, 2011), and the patients' wish to die at home would be unattainable without the work of family carers (Kinoshita et al., 2015; Hudson, 2003). Besides, when the end of life is near personal relationships satisfy existential concerns with family members and informal caregivers facilitating a process of meaning-making (Ward-Griffin et al., 2012).

However, public health palliative care extends care interactions beyond the private sphere. People with end of life care needs are active community members with roles, responsibilities, and social connections (Wright, 2003). These relationships do not cease or lose their importance with progressive frailty (Broom and Cavenagh, 2011). Palliative care has traditionally relied upon community volunteers to deliver its services and provide social connection to people with end of life care needs (Burbeck et al., 2014). Such exchanges commonly take place in hospices, hospitals, and nursing homes. Recent years have seen much mobilisation to facilitate volunteer-led interventions at home and in the community.

Various programmes that support the frail and elderly, people at the end of life and their caregivers, as well as the recently bereaved, aim to tackle social isolation and enhance their lives with purpose and meaning (Horsfall, 2018; Wegleitner et al., 2016). This is ordinarily achieved though offerings of companionship, networking, and help with practical everyday tasks, such as shopping and pet care. Community development for the end of life takes the form of informal neighbourhood support (Kellehear, 2016) that becomes invaluable to the lives of care recipients. Such programmes may be facilitated and supervised by community development workers, but they are designed in partnership with community members to reflect and represent individual and local needs.

Ambitions for Palliative and End of Life Care (National Palliative and End of Life Care Partnership, 2015) as policy and practice framework prescribes ways in which family carers and the wider community are to become integral partners in the delivery of palliative care. Despite formal recognition of the value of civic involvement, we still need to regularly revisit the philosophical foundations of palliative care to reflect upon the nature and quality of care that we provide for some of society's most vulnerable.

Risks associated with the professionalisation of palliative care are still relevant. In 1996 Bradshaw observed that the nursing profession and palliative care simultaneously underwent a shift from a culture of altruism and service to the patient towards one that prioritises professional autonomy. As a result, we witness the dominance of medical innovations, psychological/spiritual tools, and evaluation techniques over the purposes and ends that they serve. Public health palliative care may have refocused upon essential social relationships that sustain care, but the prevalence of professionalism is inhibiting a discursive negotiation of the direction of community partnerships that would help remove obstacles to inclusion and promote equality in health and wellbeing for socially disadvantaged groups.

CULTURES OF END OF LIFE CARE

Hospices and bereavement services report that ethnic minority groups underutilise their services, and express concern that certain sections of society do not receive much needed support and are effectively excluded from care (Cohen, 2008; Johnson, 2013). In their effort to promote inclusion, Compassionate Communities come up with innovative ideas. Work undertaken at St Joseph's hospice in London provides a good example of a cosmopolitan setting that embraces diversity to deliver its objectives (Sallnow et al., 2017). People with end of life care needs are befriended by volunteers who are recent migrants, with significant benefits for both parties.

However, care relationships in urban neighbourhoods occupied by close-knit ethnic minority communities with collective historical memory and distinct culture and identity, need further conceptualisation. An essential element of care provided at any stage of life is the understanding, appreciation, and fulfilment of personal, familial, and community needs. When these preconditions are not met or are partially understood, ethnic minority communities fall back upon their own support networks and mobilise grassroots care frameworks. Such a strategy is socially desirable, but we need to ensure that it is supported by public policy and practice. Community resilience should not lead to social isolation. Compassionate Cities have the potential to meet the objectives set in the Charter by aligning their work with existing culturally embedded social organisation for the end of life that responds to and meets the needs of socially disadvantaged communities.

Koffman and Higginson (2004) explain the under-utilisation of palliative care services by ethnic minority populations in terms of healthcare's lack of "cultural competency". Evans et al. (2012) challenge the usefulness of the notion of culture in explaining experiences that are arguably context-specific. Initial efforts to promote cultural sensitivity in end of life care produced concrete accounts of death rituals practiced by different ethnic minority groups (Firth, 2000; Katz, 2000; Kalsi, 1996). This is otherwise known as the "cultural factfile" approach to end of life care, which has fallen out of fashion because we know that culture is changeable and dynamic (Gunaratnam, 1997).

The objective of representing culture in end of life care may be slippery, but there is something that we could do towards firming this up. We may gain a better understanding of the social relationships that shape responses to death, dying, and bereavement to appreciate risks, vulnerabilities, and processes of resilience. McManners (1981) emphasised the need to position death related experiences within political, economic, and social structures, and within a historical context. Our approach then relies upon our capacity to practice care reflectively and relationally, with awareness of the diversity of subjective experiences that may differ or be similar and connected to our own.

Case study: Grief as a social relationship

Between 2006 and 2010, I studied bereavement among people of African-Caribbean descent in the South West of England. One of the early findings was that loss cannot be isolated from social inequalities, historic disadvantage, and racism. To capture this and the meanings attached to notions of loss and resilience, I employed an ethnographic approach to research, and spent a considerable amount of time observing care interactions and collecting documentary and audio-visual materials. To fill in a description of a dispossessed community and its end of life care relationships, I regularly visited a luncheon centre for ethnic minority senior citizens and a Pentecostal church community.

Bereavement studies commonly examine negotiations of identity stimulated by loss and grief. This is because our sense of self is heightened when we encounter difference or threat (Lawler, 2014), and grief serves to challenge our existential concerns. Research on bereavement has shifted its attention from the stages/phases of grief to the long-term meaning-making processes that accompany loss, and the continuing bonds that bereaved people maintain with the deceased (Valentine 2008; Neimeyer et al., 2006; Klass and Steffen 2017; Klass et al., 1996; Walter, 1996). However, individualistic attitudes and relative privilege in Western societies have resulted in grief literature that remains person-focused rather than engaging with the larger socio-political questions that shape end of life experiences.

Research on end of life care in the African-Caribbean community was similarly inspired by an interest in bereavement and related challenges to a coherent sense of self. However, social disadvantage inevitably puts into question the social structures that enhance death-related experiences with importance and meaning. For this purpose, I quickly turned to study the legacy of slavery, trauma, racism, and dispossession throughout history and during the post-1950s migration period in the UK. Characteristically, there was congruence between bereavement and other types of loss that refer to social conditions in participants' life narratives. Culture was shaped by understandings that originate in socio-historical experiences of racialisation, and there was investment in courage, patience, and resilience. The sentiment was encapsulated in Sylvia's comment, who stoically argued that "grief is grief", and went on to talk about life, routines, and coping upon being invited to talk about the loss of a significant other.

Studies of grief in materially deprived communities provide pathways to understanding the role of social conditions. Scheper-Hughes (1992) in her ethnographic work *Death Without Weeping* reports upon attitudes towards the loss of infant babies among impoverished mothers in Brazil. By Western standards, their behaviours contradict conceptions of motherhood. However, once placed into context, they indicate a political economy of emotions shaped by the legacy of slavery, postcolonial neglect, and the prevalence of violence. Similarly, Strange (2005) in her analysis of grief among the poor in Edwardian and Victorian England depicts experiences of loss in which coping with adversity takes priority over emotional expression. She goes on to explore silence, physical and emotional exhaustion, and continuing bonds as ways to "manage" rather than "withhold" grief. This enabled mourners "to complete the practical tasks associated with bereavement but which also provided scope for reflection, sorrow and anger in isolated moments and spaces" (Strange, 2005, p. 306).

In public perception, African-Caribbean celebrative death rituals are viewed as outlets for the expression of painful emotions, while early academic writing theorised that elaborate rituals help to overcome loss (Rosenblatt et al., 1976; Parkes et al., 1997; Eisenbruch, 1984). However, there are more sophisticated ways to interpret stoicism in marginalised communities. Rich histories of loss, dispossession, and structural inequality shape identity and provide the social capital necessary to address end of life care needs. Although research participants struggled and made no attempt to conceal their suffering, they also placed much effort into showcasing journeys of growth and empowerment that often led them to defy social stereotypes or transcend barriers to social inclusion.

Mr Ronald, an older participant, lost two children to multiple sclerosis and his sister within a matter of two years. At an in-depth informal discussion, he narrated the process of his life's reconstruction, illustrating how he employed leadership to actively promote community cohesion, challenge racial stereotypes, and better everyone's life chances. In Barbados he managed a sugar plantation and when he moved to England, he became the first black bus driver in his local city following a boycott. He has supported research on multiple sclerosis, volunteered for hospices, and set up a senior citizens association following negotiations with the council. Photographic albums and the display of memorabilia assisted him in creating a biographical account that highlights a journey through grief, stoicism, and reorganisation. His life review (Butler, 1963) constructs a legacy that unites the local African-Caribbean community based upon identification with a history that extends beyond the immediate racialised material existence and promotes social inclusion and connection to ancestry within the African-Caribbean diaspora.

HISTORICAL NARRATIVES OF LOSS AND CULTURES OF CARE

The history of slavery might be met with apprehension in British society and within the African-Caribbean community, but its legacy is crucial to our understanding of end of life care. The process of responding to loss is tainted by stereotypes and relationships that originate in colonial history.

Difference attributed to "race" served to organise political, economic, and social relationships unequally (Fenton, 1999), and justified plantocracies as totalitarian regimes. Everyday beatings, dehumanising labour, starvation, efforts to eradicate links to ancestral languages and religions, and prevention of the creation of new familial and kinship bonds served to reinforce racial stereotypes and lock slaves in what Patterson (1982) calls "social death". Analyses of death rituals performed by the enslaved, point to their centrality in representing a social status that identifies with mortality as the most common aspect of daily life (Morgan, 1997). During those moments of "liminality" (Van Gennep, 2004) when slaves were given the space to mourn their dead, they had the opportunity to connect with a higher purpose, negotiate identity, and organise protests that promoted emancipation.

The end of slavery did not necessarily signal the beginning of new social conditions. Postcolonialism perpetuated established hierarchies and continued to control the consciousness of its subjects (Fanon, 2006). Racism and subordination persisted into the post-migration period when young African-Caribbean people aspired to create new life in metropolitan England. Testimonies and first-person accounts reveal the disappointment and loss experienced by migrants for their unwelcoming reception (Phillips and Phillips, 1998).

At this stage, death rituals came once again to represent the lived experience of social exclusion in British society. Valeria, a community leader and key informant, testified that funerals at this time in history were mournful and reflected the mood of a community that had regained trust and allowed itself to re-invest in a special bond with Motherland England, only to be rejected. End of life care was conveniently appropriated and reconstructed to reinvent bonds and promote resilience amidst fragmentation and disenfranchised loss that lacks social recognition.

Although I carried out interviews to extract bereavement narratives, my observations produced insights on death and dying, as well as ageing. Social disadvantage creates the preconditions for the development of support networks that respond to all end of life care needs. A bereaved person would have been supported throughout their caring journey as their loved one was dying, and there are processes in place to provide caring environments for people in old age.

Community organisation for the end of life is driven by an ethical commitment towards people who have lived a hard life, migrated to better the livelihood of their children, and advance their community. It is believed that they deserve to live and die with dignity in old age. This is especially the case when trust in equality is questionable and civil society cannot guarantee a good death. It is a reciprocal responsibility of the young and able towards the frail and elderly to create a harmonious and cohesive social environment supportive of the end of life within a protective and nurturing community.

A RESILIENT COMMUNITY

Historical experience makes grief part of the cultural outlook with which African-Caribbean people live and survive. All loss, including bereavement, is met with acceptance. However, resilience is the product of vulnerability. Women and men alike of various age groups see in their bereavement the social conditions of their existence, whether that involves a life lost prematurely, a separation or divorce prior to death, a life of hard labour, poverty, and migration, separation from biological parents or people that took parenting roles, lack of opportunities for social mobility, and encounters with racism. Bereavement presents a unique opportunity for review, change, and repositioning in social life. And although there is adaptive strength in this response, there might also be a need for emotional care that has been neglected. For this reason, most research participants found release in the interview encounter.

Bereavement is also subject to personal relationships and family structures. Historically, family organisation in the African-Caribbean experience represents a cultural resource responsive to crisis (Whitehead, 1978; Gordon, 1997). Its adaptive strength protects the orphaned, dispossessed, the frail and elderly, the dying, and the bereaved, even when their prioritisation compromises societal expectations. Tasha, for example, was raised by her grandparents in Jamaica before she joined her parents in England. As a teenager she moved in with her uncle and auntie who she referred to as "parents". It is their loss that she grieved in her adult life.

Taking responsibility, embracing the value of reciprocity, and supporting others even when one is confronted with loss and bereavement, provides opportunities for social recognition and positive identification. Social cohesion is realised within adaptive repositioning to constant dislocation, disruption of collective memory, mortality, and violence in everyday life, as well as in irregular family and kin relations that become responsive to loss. Identifications in this context are hybrid (Gilroy, 1993; Hall, 1996) renditions of hegemonic ideals set by the dominant culture during colonial history that serve to upset and transform social order. Despite internal variation, familiarity with loss, appreciation of the precarity of social life, and cultivated stoicism brings the community together in support of those perceived to be vulnerable. In this space, compassion is heartfelt and unconditional.

African-Caribbean women exhibit qualities of maturity and independence and remain active in productive economy. All their efforts are ultimately directed towards supporting vulnerable family members and promoting community resilience. Research participants demonstrated unique understanding of grief's psychology either in the form of lay knowledge and/or professional competence. They applied their skills to mentor the young and support older people in professional and voluntary roles, and very often both. This is a form of communitarian work that involves personal and political investment, for no material sense of reward or benefit – other than a kind of pay it forward orientation. These are communities that have been underserved, while those with necessary social, cultural, and arguably economic capital make themselves available to firstly recognise, and then protect and develop their community.

Bereavement then comes as realisation that they need to get out of a limited mindset, gain in self-esteem, recover from physical and emotional exhaustion, and meet the potential of their strength and wisdom. Tasha acknowledged that "all the -isms are still there. We need to free our minds from mental slavery. I'm not good enough, I'm black, you got to move out of this. Once you get out, others will follow". The meaning-making process following loss represents a form of working politics by stealth, and through reframing one's personal and collective identity within areas that require improvement. Knowing that to support others, they need to first accumulate personal resources, African-Caribbean women exercise self-care, redefine priorities, and/or pursue a different career path, training opportunities, or educational qualifications. In this way, they unwittingly offer role-modelling to younger generations and pursue transformational causes intended to emancipate a marginalised population.

PERSONAL NARRATIVES OF LOSS

Loss compromises personal resilience and suspends learned resistance to risk, even if temporarily. African-Caribbean people have developed in the course of history stoical responses to grief to avert attracting violence or insult at times of heightened vulnerability (Morgan, 1997). Poverty and the need to keep up with responsibilities and maintain economic productivity, provide additional incentives to remain centred, while continuing to grieve. Mrs Monica described grief as an inner state of troublesome emotions that bereaved people make every effort to conceal. A metaphor comparing grief to the experience of wearing shoes a size too small, was employed to convey the indescribable suffering caused by loss that leaves hidden marks:

> …it's one of them pain that you cannot share that kind of pain with anybody…It's like when you have got a shoe that is hurting your feet and you can't find the money to get yourself a new pair of shoes, a bigger size. You've got to keep wearing those shoes until you have a little corn on your toe. Have you ever been though that when you had a little corn your toe because your shoe is too tight? You try to walk stylish because you don't want anybody to see you are hurting but, you know…it's the same with losses.

Structural inequality serves to contain but also compound grief among African-Caribbean men who experience masculinity in contradictory terms. In line with Connel's (2012) gender hierarchy, men that have historically been enslaved and therefore excluded from status gained in ownership relations, do not straightforwardly attain the ideal of hegemonic masculinity. If they continue to encounter glass ceilings when they attempt to access leadership roles, they will identify with the loss of a subordinate masculinity. In this space, there are multiple possibilities of existing, all of which feature the interweaving causal effects of disenfranchised grief and bereavement. Poverty and racialised disadvantage have a compromising effect upon personal relations that cost intimate bonds, and occasionally lives lost in adversity.

Mr Anderson aimed high in his career within the Royal Air Force, but institutional racism contained his ambition. His frequent postings undermined harmony within his household, while his seniors announced that they could no longer keep a man with a disconcerted wife under their line of management. His marriage ended in divorce and in his old age, Mr Anderson was emotionally isolated. After years of progressively deteriorating health, his former wife died, while his daughter had since become estranged. Our multiple conversations allowed him to join the fragmented pieces of his life story together into a coherent narrative. Recognition of the value his ex-wife added to his life, allowed him a renewed sense of self.

John grew up in the UK in the 1960s and 1970s within a society that set unrealistic expectations via a meritocratic education system that stereotyped him as underachiever. His own mother adopted a punitive approach to his upbringing and would often pre-empt that he would "never turn to anything good". To escape judgement, John joined a deviant urban subculture. The death of his younger brother in a tragic car accident, a year after he had been severely beaten and incapacitated by a rival gang, contributed to John's fundamental review of the methods and practices by which he achieved recognition. Following his release from a convent where he isolated for a year, he assumed an active role within his religious community, engaged in charitable activity, and tried to reach out to others who had lost their way. At the same time, he took an interest and started studying spirituality and history to reflect upon and understand his experience.

Joseph was rejected by his family and African-Caribbean community for being gay. Racialised rejection also became a theme in his interactions within the gay community. For years, he lived in the "wilderness", growing progressively more accustomed and at the same time indifferent to insults of bigotry and racialised harassment. When he met his Afro-Indian-Carib grandmother, he was pleasantly surprised at her expressions of unconditional acceptance and "love". Their relationship, that lasted until her death in old age, gave him inspiration and strength to create a professional profile with which he is helping African-Caribbean gay men to accept themselves and live healthy lifestyles.

The web of social dimensions associated with loss and grief in the African-Caribbean experience call for a response that supports cohesion as a viable way to better health and wellbeing, as well as greater equality and representation in society. It has been established that poverty and racism cause ill health and are responsible for early mortality (Barry and Yuill, 2016), while COVID-19 has highlighted the mechanisms under increased exposure to risk affecting ethnic minority populations (Platt and Warwick, 2020). Public health approaches to end of life care acknowledge that social exclusion is detrimental to health and aim to alleviate its effects among people with end of life care needs. Compassionate Cities specifically target marginalised communities for being more susceptible to the effects of social isolation.

What remains to be observed is that vulnerable communities already organise for eventualities known to compromise health and wellbeing. Unconditional participation in the African-Caribbean community remains an option to anyone – outsiders included – who needs support and care in crisis. Centred around a place of religious worship or a council-funded organisation that supports ethnic minority senior citizens, members of the African-Caribbean community find opportunities to set up organically nurtured networks of compassionate care. Professional roles are complemented by voluntary involvement, while both are deployed within a grassroots framework of care to address needs defined locally.

Valeria, as community leader, community development worker, and business owner runs the Senior Citizens Ethnic Minority Association in her locality, maintains a catering company, organises funerary rituals, and gives free advice on preparations for death and dying. In her free time, she pays home visits to provide companionship and practical support to bereaved and elderly community members. Valeria has "inherited" the leadership of the African-Caribbean community from Mr Ronald. Her team of predominantly female community champions collectively act as guardians of a system that sustains personalised care and meets subjective need in order to build cohesion and counteract social disadvantage.

Upon being invited to a funeral, I contemplated that I would act discrete within my role of food service. However, I soon realised that an invitation to a funeral party is open to everyone who is willing to join in the celebrations of a life "well lived". It was an ordinary family that hosted an event for a diverse crowd they were not necessarily acquainted with. Young people were included in the ritual, and marijuana smoking was tolerated in the backyard. While the bereaved family was greeting visitors arriving to pay their respects, a very diverse group of mourners was drinking, dancing, and embracing in the room next door. In this respect, the meaning of celebratory rituals is found in the role they play in reinforcing social bonds, promoting inclusion, and recreating life anew.

INTER-CULTURAL COLLABORATION IN PALLIATIVE AND END OF LIFE CARE

Health policy has reoriented towards the provision of care in community settings, and interprofessional partnerships are essential in the implementation of related directions. However, Marmot (2015) warns that such developments cannot address the inequalities responsible for producing differential health outcomes across the population. To bridge discrepancy in life expectancy, we need to tackle the "causes of causes" such as racialisation and the uneven distribution of wealth within and across societies.

Although it is beyond the remit of public health end of life care to address such considerations, Compassionate Cities can have an equalising effect should they work with the vulnerabilities that affect local communities. If related initiatives fall short of their aims and objectives, it could be attributed to the terms and conditions that come with funding. The prioritisation of evidence-based innovation and professional competency in the delivery of support and care for citizens can withdraw decision-making from local leadership. In reality, compassion is enhanced with purpose when minority and grassroots approaches to the practice of care are represented within models and lead community interventions. This is because greater social integration can improve health and wellbeing even at the presence of causes that contribute to health inequalities. Cuba and Costa Rica, for example, countries that despite poverty concentrate significant social capital around health and wellbeing, exhibit comparable levels of life expectancy with the world's superpower, the United States of America, where income disparities are extreme (Barry and Yuill, 2016, p. 78).

What remains to be considered is the meaning of compassion and practices that cultivate it. Our preceding discussion on the role of culture in end of life care, precludes that understandings of subjective suffering containing the essence of compassion cannot follow a formulae defined by culturally prescriptive practices. Analyses of contextual circumstances and social conditions provide a window to the lived experience of marginalised communities, their risks, vulnerabilities, and end of life care needs. However, the accessibility of such knowledge is limited unless simplified.

The Sociological Imagination (Mills, 1959) provides a method of inquiry that taps upon "personal troubles" of biography in order to reflect upon "public issues" of history and structure. Within any given society we should be able to relate to another's experience by observing our own, because our realities remain inextricable intertwined, even when they diverge. Modernisation has not been exclusive of antagonistic conflict, while increasing familiarity in global societies contrasts our differences (see Martell, 2017, pp. 73–88). However, inter-relatedness provides an advantageous perspective from which we can estrange what we take for granted, take distance, and examine the mundane and yet remarkable experiences of everyday life under new light and from the vantage point of multiple and differing narratives.

Progressively and as if connecting pieces in a puzzle, by following up clues and asking questions, we can succeed at building a story about subjective experience that sets new directions for practice. This is what Back (2007) calls artful and attentive listening that allows access to conceptual understanding even when our own story implicates and is part of the evolving description. In fact, Butler (2004) argues that it is necessary to come to terms with our own precarity and grieve our losses, personal and collective, if we are to acknowledge the universality of loss and work towards an egalitarian peace-building politics. With reference to the post 9/11 American society, she observes how denial of grief within the nation and failure to acknowledge its role in the Middle East, justified a defensive response that produced more war and human casualties.

As we move towards a cosmopolitan order we become less reliant upon categorical thinking in order to understand our lives and practices. However, historical trauma, "discrimination and racist acts of inhumanity in the past whose effects have been so damaging on a group of people that requires generations to heal" (Barry and Yuill, 2016, p. 125), continue to undermine social cohesion and divide communities. At the same time, extreme disparities in power and status, and uneven distribution of wealth perpetuate disadvantage and create an array of social problems (Wilkinson and Pickett, 2010).

In everyday life, and in professional/interprofessional practice, it becomes increasingly important to be responsive to temporal identifications. There are emancipatory possibilities in this direction, but unless we reflect upon experiences that construct us vulnerable, fragile, and ephemeral we will perpetuate cycles of expansion followed by defensive retraction. Negotiations of inter-related experiences of suffering, loss, and grief do not only find verbal expression. Compassionate Cities, and indeed all citizens, can reflect upon their own gains and losses to gradually allow a challenge to the hierarchical order of care relationships. This is a gesture of commitment to communities that have been underserved, to their inclusion, cohesion, and improving wellbeing.

Compassionate Cities work with all end of life care experiences, including bereavement, and make it a priority to support marginalised communities. Cultural engagement paves the way to this end. Action 10 states that "all services and policies will demonstrate an understanding of how diversity shapes the experience of ageing, dying, death, loss and care" (Kellehear, 2016). However, our understanding of processes that shape cultural responses to loss and determine the formation of care relationships goes beyond policy development. Intersubjective communication needs to be integrated or acknowledged, actively and discursively, within systems and processes of support – a complex endeavour that permeates and transforms the foundations of social, ethnic, and civic relations. Compassion in end of life care implies presence in another person's suffering. This is attainable even when perceptions of social reality diverge because we bond upon an ethical paradox that prioritises cohesion and peace-building despite contradictory relationality (Butler, 2020).

KEY POINTS

- The public health approach to palliative care, exemplified through the Compassionate Communities and Compassionate Cities movements, aims to support the natural processes of death, dying, and bereavement within the community. This is to some extent a reaction against the medicalisation and professionalisation of death and dying.
- Communities have diverse practices relating to death, dying, bereavement, and caring, which have evolved over time in response to social conditions.
- Meaningful engagement between communities and palliative care services requires not simply knowledge about these practices but also understanding of the historical, political, and socio-economic background to them.
- Greater understanding will contribute towards greater integration, more equality of access, and better representation of communities and their needs within end of life care services.

REFERENCES

Abel, J, Kingston, H, Scally, A, et al. (2018) Reducing emergency hospital admissions: a population health complex intervention of an enhanced model of primary care and compassionate communities. *British Journal of General Practice*, 68(676), e803–e810.

Aries, P (1974) *Western attitudes toward death: from the middle ages to the present*. Johns Hopkins University Press, Baltimore.

Back, L (2007) *The art of listening*. Bloomsbury, London.

Barry, A-M, Yuill, C (2016) *Understanding the sociology of health*. 4th ed. SAGE, Los Angeles.

Bradshaw, A (1996) The spiritual dimension of hospice: the secularisation of an ideal. *Social Science and Medicine*, 43(3), 409–419.

Broom, A, Cavenagh, J (2011) On the meanings and experiences of living and dying in an Australian hospice. *Health*, 15(1), 96–111.

Burbeck, R, Candy, B, Low, J, Rees, R (2014) Understanding the role of the volunteer in specialist palliative care: a systematic review and thematic synthesis of qualitative studies. *BMC Palliative Care*, 13, 3.

Butler, J (2004) *Precarious life: the powers of mourning and violence*. Verso, London.

Butler, RN (1963) The life review: an interpretation of reminiscence in the aged. *Psychiatry*, 26(1), 65–76. doi: 10.1080/00332747.1963.11023339

Butler, J (2020) *The force of non-violence: an ethico-political bind.* London, Verso.

Cohen, LL (2008) Racial/ethnic disparities in hospice care: a systematic review. *Journal of Palliative Medicine*, 11(5). doi: 10.1089/jpm.2007.0216

Collins, A, Brown, JEH, Mills, J, Philip, J (2020) The impact of public health palliative care interventions on health system outcomes: A systematic review. *Palliative Medicine*, 1–13: doi.org/10.1177/0269216320981722

Connel, R (2012) Gender, health and theory: conceptualising the issue in local and world perspective. *Social Science and Medicine*, 74(11), 1675–1683.

Costa-Requena, G, Espinosa Val, MC, Cristofol, R (2015) Caregiver burden in end of life care: advanced cancer and final stage of dementia. *Palliative and Supportive Care*, 13(3), 583–589.

Eisenbruch, M (1984) Cross-cultural aspects of bereavement II: ethnic and cultural variations in the development of bereavement practices. *Culture, Medicine and Psychiatry*, 8(4), 315–347.

Evans, N, Menaca, A, Andrew, EVW, et al. (2012) Systematic review of the primary research on minority ethnic groups and end-of-life care from the United Kingdom. *Journal of Pain and Symptom Management*, 43(2), 261–286.

Fanon, F (2006) Racism and culture. In A Haddour (ed.) *The fanon reader.* Pluto Press, London.

Fenton, S (1999) *Ethnicity: racism, class and culture.* Macmillan Press, London.

Firth, S (2000) Approaches to death in Hindu and Sikh communities in Britain. In D Dickenson, M Johnson, JS Katz (eds.) *Death, dying and bereavement.* SAGE, London.

Fried, TR, Bradley, EH, O'Leary, JR, Byers, AL (2004) Unmet desire for caregiver-patient communication and increased caregiver burden. *Journal of the American Geriatrics Society*, 53(1), 59–65.

Gilroy, P (1993) *The black atlantic: modernity and double consciousness.* Harvard University Press, Cambridge, UK.

Glajchen, M (2004) The emerging role and needs of family caregivers in cancer care. *The Journal of Supportive Oncology*, 2(2), 145–155.

Gordon, ET (1997) Cultural politics of black masculinity. *Transforming Anthropology*, 6(1–2), 36–53.

Gunaratnam, Y (1997) Culture is not enough: a critique of multiculturalism in palliative care. In D Field, J Hockey, N Small (eds.) *Death, gender and ethnicity.* Routledge, London.

Hall, S (1996) New ethnicities. In D Morley and K-H Chen, (eds.) *Critical dialogues in cultural studies.* Routledge, London.

Hebert, RS, Schultz, R (2006) Caregiving at the end of life. *Journal of Palliative Medicine*, 9(5), 1174–1187.

Holt-Lunstad, J, Smith, TB (2012) Social relationships and mortality. *Social and Personality Psychology Compass*, 6(1), 41–53.

Horsfall, D (2018) Developing compassionate communities in Australia through collective caregiving: a qualitative study exploring network-centred care and the role of the end of life sector. *Annals of Palliative Medicine*, 7(Suppl 2), S42–S51.

Hudson, P (2003) Home-based support for palliative care families: challenges and recommendations. *Medical Journal of Australia*, 179, s35–s37.

Hudson, P, Payne, S (2011) Family caregivers and palliative care: current status and agenda for the future. *Journal of Palliative Medicine*, 14(7). doi: 10.1089/jpm.2010.0413

Johnson, K (2013) Racial and ethnic disparities in palliative care. *Journal of Palliative Medicine*, 16(11), 1329–1334.

Kalsi, S (1996) Change and continuity in the funeral rituals of Sikhs in Britain. In G Howarth, P Jupp (eds.) *Contemporary issues in the sociology of death, dying and disposal.* Macmillan, Basingstoke.

Katz, J (2000) Jewish perspectives on death, dying and bereavement. In D Dickenson, M Johnson, JS Katz (eds.) *Death, dying and bereavement*. SAGE, London.

Kellehear, A (1999) *Health promoting palliative care*. Oxford University Press, Melbourne.

Kellehear, A (2005) *Compassionate cities: public health and end-of-life care*. Routledge, New York.

Kellehear, A (2016) Compassionate city charter: inviting the cultural and social sectors into end of life care. In K Wegleitner, K Heimerl, A Kellehear (eds.) *Compassionate communities: case studies from Britain and Europe*. Routledge, London, pp. 76–87.

Kinoshita, H, Maeda, I, Morita, T, et al. (2015) Place of death and differences in the quality of patient death and dying and caregiver burden. *Journal of Clinical Oncology*, 33(4), 357–363.

Klass, D, Silverman, PR, Nickman, S (1996) *Continuing bonds: new understandings of grief*. New York: Taylor & Francis.

Klass, D, Steffen, EM (2017) *Continuing bonds in bereavement: new directions for research and practice*. New York: Routledge.

Koffman, J, Higginson, IJ (2004) Dying to be home? Preferred location of death of first-generation black Caribbean and native born white patients in the United Kingdom. *Palliative and Supportive Care*, 7, 628–636.

Lawler, S (2014) *Identity: sociological perspectives*. 2nd ed. Polity Press, Cambridge.

Marmot, M (2015) *The health gap: the challenge of an unequal world*. Bloomsbury, London.

Martell, L (2017) *The sociology of globalisation*. 2nd ed. Cambridge, Polity Press.

McManners, J (1981) *Death and the enlightenment: changing attitudes to death in eighteenth-century France*. Oxford University Press, Oxford.

Mills, CW (1959) *The sociological imagination*. Oxford University Press, New York.

Morgan, PD (1997) The cultural implications of the Atlantic slave trade: African regional origins, American destinations and new world developments. *Slavery and Abolition*, 18(1), 122–145.

National Palliative and End of Life Care Partnership (2015) *Ambitions for palliative and end and of life care: a national framework for local action 2015–2020*. http://endoflif ecareambitions.org.uk/wp-content/uploads/2015/09/Ambitions-for-Palliative-and-End -of-Life-Care.pdf

Neimeyer, RA, Baldwin, SA, Gillies, J (2006) Continuing bonds and reconstructing meaning: mitigating complications in bereavement. *Death Studies*, 30(8), 715–738.

Parkes, CM, Laungani, P, Young, B (1997) *Death and bereavement across cultures*. Routledge, New York.

Patterson, O (1982) *Slavery and social death: a comparative study*. President and Fellows of Harvard College, Cambridge, MA.

Phillips, M, Phillips, T (1998) *Windrush: the irresistible rise of multi-racial Britain*. Harper Collins Publishers, London.

Platt, L, Warwick, R (2020) *Are some ethnic groups more vulnerable to COVID-19 than others?* Institute for Fiscal Studies. https://www.ifs.org.uk/inequality/chapter/are-some -ethnic-groups-more-vulnerable-to-covid-19-than-others/ (accessed 18 November 2020).

Rosenblatt, PC, Walsh, R, Jackson, D (1976) *Grief and mourning in cross-cultural perspective*. HRAP Press, Washington, DC.

Sallnow, L, Richardson, H, Murray, S, Kellehear, A (2017) Understanding the impact of a new public health approach to end-of-life care: a qualitative study of a community led intervention. *The Lancet*, 389(S88). doi: 10.1016/S0140-6736(17)30484-1

Scheper-Hughes, N (1992) *Death without weeping: the violence of everyday life in Brazil*. University of California Press, California.

Strange, J-M (2005) *Death, drief and poverty in Britain, 1870–1914*. Cambridge University Press, Cambridge.

Valentine, C (2008) *Bereavement narratives: continuing bonds in the twenty-first century.* Routledge, London.

Van Gennep, A (2004) *The rites of passage.* Routledge, London.

Waldrop, DP, Kramer, BJ, Skretny, JA, Milch, RA, Finn, W (2005) Final transitions: family caregiving at the end of life. *Journal of Palliative Medicine,* 8(3), 623–637.

Walter, T (1996) A new model of grief: bereavement and biography. *Mortality,* 1, 7–25.

Ward-Griffin, C, McWilliam, CL, Oudshoorn, A (2012) Relational experiences of family caregivers providing home-based end-of-life care. *Journal of Family Nursing,* 18(4), 491–516.

Wegleitner, K, Heimerl, K, Kellehear, A (2016) *Compassionate communities: case studies from Britain and Europe.* Routledge, London.

Whitehead, TL (1978) Residence, kinship and mating as survival strategies: a West Indian example. *Journal of Marriage and Family,* 40(4), 817–828.

Wilkinson, R, Pickett, K (2010) *The spirit level: why equality is better for everyone.* Penguin, London.

Wright, K (2003) Relationships with death: the terminally ill talk about dying. *Journal of Marital and Family Therapy,* 29(4), 439–454.

CHAPTER 9

Collaboration in palliative care

Global perspectives

....

Dave Roberts, Zipporah Ali, and Brigid Sirengo

OUTLINE

Palliative care is an internationally recognised area of specialist practice with a global reach. The World Health Organisation (WHO) has provided a definition that is accepted globally and provides a basis for international collaboration:

> Palliative care is an approach that improves the quality of life of patients and their families facing the problems associated with life-threatening illness, through the prevention and relief of suffering by means of early identification and impeccable assessment and treatment of pain and other problems, physical, psychosocial and spiritual.
>
> *(WHO 2002)*

The WHO has adopted a Palliative Care Public Health Strategy, which aims to integrate palliative care services into health care and has the following features: appropriate national policies, drug availability (particularly opioids), education of health care workers and the public, and developing palliative care services throughout society with community empowerment (Stjernsward, 2007). This chapter explores how this approach has been applied in different countries and settings globally.

BACKGROUND: GLOBAL PALLIATIVE CARE

In 2011, 115 of the world's 234 countries (58%) had some form of palliative care services, an increase of 9% from 2006 as 21 countries developed new services. If

DOI: 10.4324/9781351113472-9

services in development are included, the percentage rises to 68% (Lynch et al., 2013), and it is likely that it has continued to grow globally.

However, this is far from a universal growth in palliative care. Growth has been greatest, unsurprisingly, in the high income countries where resources are most freely available. These developed countries share several characteristics:

- A strong and effectively implemented national palliative care policy framework.
- High levels of public spending on healthcare services.
- Extensive palliative care training resources for general and specialised medical workers.
- Generous subsidies to reduce the financial burden of palliative care on patients.
- Wide availability of opioid analgesics.
- Strong public awareness of palliative care.

(The Economist 2015)

Countries without these essential elements will make slower progress but there have been promising developments nonetheless. These often involve local solutions to local problems but are based on universal transferable principles of palliative care. Examples of significant progress in lower and middle income countries include Panama, where a primary care model of palliative care is becoming established, Mongolia, which has seen rapid growth in hospice facilities and education, and Uganda, which has made significant progress in the availability of opioid medication (The Economist 2015).

The progress towards developing palliative care services globally can been charted through surveys conducted by European institutions in collaboration with local partners (Table 9.1).

WORKING ACROSS INTERNATIONAL BOUNDARIES

Much of the development of palliative care globally has been achieved on the basis of international collaborations. Palliative care professionals and academics from developed countries can support colleagues in the developing world to establish and progress palliative care services. This can be by providing mentorship, education, material assistance, and by collaboration on joint research and development projects. There are different strategic approaches to this form of international collaboration. At its most simple level, it may involve professionals with expertise in palliative care visiting other countries where it is less well developed. This may initially involve observation, but move on to fund raising, education, and sharing of expertise. The following case study includes an account taken from the blog of one British nurse visiting the emerging palliative care services in Cambodia.

Table 9.1 Global surveys of palliative care

Publication	Institution(s)
Wright, M, Wood, J, Lynch, T, Clark, D (2008) Mapping Levels of Palliative Care Development: a Global View. Journal of Pain and Symptom Management, 35(5), pp. 469–85.	International Observatory on End of Life Care, Lancaster University.
Lynch T, Connor S, Clark D (2013) Mapping levels of palliative care development: A global update. Journal of Pain and Symptom Management; 45(6), pp. 1094–1106.	International Observatory on End of Life Care, Lancaster University.
Centeno C, Pons JJ, Lynch T, Donea O, Rocafort J, Clark D (2013) EAPC Atlas of Palliative Care in Europe 2013 - Cartographic Edition. Milan: EAPC Press.	EAPC Task Force on the Development of Palliative Care in Europe. ATLANTES Research Group, Institute for Culture and Society, University of Navarra, Spain. The University of Glasgow.
Rhee JY, Luyirika E, Namisango E, Powell RA, Garralda E, Pons JJ, de Lima L, Centeno C (2017) APCA Atlas of Palliative Care in Africa. IAHPC Press.	African Palliative Care Association. Arnhold Institute for Global Health at the Icahn School of Medicine at Mount Sinai. International Association for Hospice and Palliative Care (IAHPC). ATLANTES Research Program at the Institute for Culture and Society at the University of Navarra.
Osman H, Rihan A, Garralda E, Rhee JY, Pons JJ, de Lima L, Tfayli A, Centeno C (2017) Atlas of Palliative Care in the Eastern Mediterranean Region. Houston: IAHPC Press.	Lebanese Center for Palliative Care – Balsam. ATLANTES Research Program at the Institute for Culture and Society, University of Navarra, Spain. International Association for Hospice and Palliative Care (IAHPC).
Arias-Casais N, Garralda E, Rhee JY, Lima L de, Pons JJ, Clark D, Hasselaar J, Ling J, Mosoiu D, Centeno C (2019) EAPC Atlas of Palliative Care in Europe 2019. Vilvoorde: EAPC Press.	European Association for Palliative Care (EAPC). eATLANTES Research Programme, Institute for Culture and Society, and the University of Navarra (UNAV). International Association for Hospice and Palliative Care (IAHPC).
Worldwide Hospice Palliative Care Alliance. Global Atlas of Palliative Care 2nd edn (2020) Worldwide Hospice Palliative Care Alliance. London.	Worldwide Hospice Palliative Care Alliance (WHPCA). World Health Organization (WHO).

Case study 1: Cambodia – Isolated palliative care provision

Cambodia is still recovering from a period of civil war and foreign occupation in the 1970s and 80s. In spite of some economic growth, there is widespread poverty, corruption and limited access to educational opportunities. The overall health infrastructure is fragile and under resourced. Palliative care services show an isolated pattern of provision, with funding that is heavily donor dependent, limited availability of morphine, and a small number of palliative care services in relation to the size of the population (WHPCA 2020). Such provision as exists is mainly based in urban centres and run by charities (Pav et al., 2015).

> The patient, a woman in her fifties, has been referred by "word of mouth" to the team. Diagnosed two years ago with uterine cancer, she now has metastases to her clavicle and significant problems with pain. As with many patients, she stopped chemotherapy because the family could no longer afford it and was discharged from oncology services... She has a large swelling on her clavicle – a metastasis from a uterine primary cancer. It is affecting her voice and her breathing, and she has developed numbness in her right arm. There is no option for palliative radiotherapy. She says she feels breathless all of the time. Sometimes the swelling obstructs her swallowing as well... She is tachycardic and tachypnoeic.
>
> The team carry a bag of medications. Supplies are scarce and sometimes decisions need to be made based more on practicalities and cost than clinical evidence. For example, I am told about a patient with cranial metastases who needed to take twelve prednisolone tablets because that was the cheapest way to provide the therapeutic dose of corticosteroid. Medications are purchased from overseas as this is around ten times cheaper than buying from local pharmacists. There are also significant problems in regulation and quality of local drugs, and particular concerns about opioids.
>
> *(Green, 2019)*

As you can see from this account, being alongside palliative care services in the developing world can be a culture shock for visitors. Conditions overall may be very different and challenging, and the availability of services, like radiotherapy, of personnel, and of drugs, is far less than what is available in developed countries. It can be particularly shocking to see how unaffordable drug treatments are when there is no universal health system or even insurance. Drugs may be even more expensive than in the developed countries.

Poor or variable access to strong opioids continues to be probably the single biggest obstacle to palliative care in the area, a result of stringent governmental regulation and opioidophobia (Cleary et al., 2013). In Cambodia, a maximum of seven days' supply is given at a time, which means that access can be problematic for the 90% of the population who live in remote rural areas. Essentially this means that without changes to high level policy, fundraising will not widen access to effective pain relief particularly for the poorest in the region.

There are many challenges to face in developing palliative care in resource-poor countries and settings. Factors that can restrict the development of palliative care include

- Lack of adequate resources, or overreliance on donor funding.
- Myths about opioid use or restrictive laws and regulation of drugs.
- Shortages of suitably qualified staff and lack of education programmes.
- Poor transport and infrastructure, neglect of more remote areas.
- Overcentralised and bureaucratic systems.

(De Lima, Hamzah 2004)

However, these may be overcome if there are key people who serve as champions of palliative care, if there are international partners who can give mentorship and material aid, and if local government bodies can be brought on board to support developments. The following describes how successful collaborations, both international and national, have led to the development of palliative care in one country, Kenya.

KENYA: THE DEVELOPMENT OF PALLIATIVE CARE PRACTICE AND POLICY

Kenya is a developing country in East Africa, and its capital, Nairobi, is one of the most important cities in Africa. In Kenya, the main focus of palliative care is on HIV and AIDS and cancer. There were 1.2 million AIDS-related deaths in sub-Saharan Africa in 2012 (UN, 2013). During the same period, there were 0.5 million deaths from cancer. Whilst HIV infections are now declining in Africa, cancer rates are rising: they are expected to grow by 400% over the next 50 years (Harding, Higginson 2005).

The incidence of non-communicable diseases account for more than 50% of total hospital admissions and over 55% of hospital deaths (Kenya National Strategy for the Prevention and Control of Non Communicable Diseases 2015–2020). Most patients are in advanced stages of disease and require palliative care. Even for those with an early diagnosis, palliative care is important since the majority will not be able to either access or afford treatment aimed at cure. Therefore, there is a great need to expand palliative care services, bring these services close to those who need them and to integrate palliative care services into the public health care system.

Palliative care has grown in East Africa at an impressive rate. Uganda and Kenya, both countries with high rates of HIV infection, have achieved a degree of integration of palliative care with mainstream health services that is comparable with many European countries. However, whilst there has been considerable development of services, actual provision on the ground shows large disparities, and there are considerable differences from countries with more advanced palliative care. This is illustrated by the rate of palliative care services to population: in Kenya in 2011 there were 44 services (one service for every 1,000,000 people), in the UK, 1295 services (one service for every 50,000 people) (Lynch et al., 2013). By 2017, in Kenya this had grown to 1.5 services per 1,000,000 people (Rhee et al., 2017).

The first case from Kenya (Case study 2) illustrates how collaborative working between national partners within Kenya, and funding bodies from outside the country, have developed an integrated model of palliative care, consistent with the public health model advocated by WHO, with national policies, education, and drug availability (Stjernsward, 2007).

Case study 2: Integrating palliative care into the Kenyan public health care system

Kenya Hospices and Palliative Care Association (KEHPCA), the national organisation for hospice and palliative care in Kenya, has continuously advocated for scaling up hospice and palliative care services; palliative care education of both health care and non-health care workers; public awareness; and research in palliative care. In 2010, palliative care in Kenya was solely provided by the few existing hospices. There was limited availability, as these were not widely spread across the country. KEHPCA recognised the need for palliative care services to be integrated into the health care system if more patients and families were to benefit from these services. The association approached the Ministry of Health (MoH), and made presentations to the relevant heads of the different departments in the ministry, making a strong case for the need of integration. In 2010, the director of medical services at the MoH wrote to 11 provincial hospitals to ask them to work with KEHPCA to initiate palliative care services.

Funding was made available to KEHPCA through the former Diana Princess of Wales Memorial Fund (DPWMF) and The True Colours Trust, both UK organisations. Under this project, these funding organisations worked closely with the African Palliative Care Association (APCA) and KEHPCA to integrate palliative care into 11 provincial hospitals. KEHPCA's first activity was advocacy and creating awareness at institutional levels, involving visits to hospital management teams in each site and conducting educational sessions. KEHPCA organised five-day training courses for 20 Health Care Professionals (HCPs) in each hospital, followed by a three day clinical placement in a nearby hospice. A total of 220 HCPs were trained over a period of one year using a national curriculum developed by KEHPCA and adapted by the MoH.

Each hospital selected a team leader and assigned one to two nurses to work closely with KEHPCA to set up a palliative care unit (PCU) within the hospital. Rooms were identified for the team to use. However, patients were seen within the hospital wards if they were inpatients. The trained HCPs were able to identify patients who needed palliative care and refer them to the PCU. The palliative care teams participated in ward rounds as a part of the decision-making teams. On discharge, the team aimed to link patients to a local hospice, where there was one, or patients could continue to receive outpatient services at the PCU in the hospital.

11 provincial hospitals successfully integrated palliative care within their institutions as a result of this project, serving over 30,000 patients. Of the 220 HCPs trained, many have gone on to take a higher diploma or a degree in palliative care, thus strengthening the hospitals' capacity to become centres of excellence in service provision and education. The 11 hospitals are now used as clinical and mentorship sites for other hospitals which want to integrate palliative care.

As a result of the success of this project, it was extended to 30 other hospitals across the country. Over 45 hospitals now have integrated palliative care services (PCUs) and 11 of these are now centres of excellence. Over 600 health care providers have been trained and approximately 60,000 patients have benefited from these services. Oral morphine, through support from American Cancer Society and the Danish International Development Agency (DANIDA), is now available in the hospital palliative care units.

Looking at this picture of success, it is instructive to consider the factors that have contributed to it. The survey conducted by Wright et al., published in 2008, established a model for understanding the development of palliative care within a country. This identified four levels of development: 1 no known activity; 2 capacity building; 3 localised provision; and 4 approaching integration. At the time of this original survey, Kenya had achieved level 4, approaching integration, along with two other African countries: Uganda and South Africa. Following the later survey in 2011 (Lynch et al., 2013), the model had been further refined to include two subdivisions of levels 3 and 4. By this time, six African countries were in level 4, and Kenya attained level 4a, preliminary integration. The criteria associated with a stage of preliminary integration into mainstream service provision (level 4a) include (Lynch et al., 2013):

- The development of a critical mass of palliative care activism in a number of locations.
- A variety of palliative care providers and types of services.
- Awareness of palliative care on the part of health professionals and local communities.
- The availability of morphine and some other strong pain-relieving drugs.
- Limited impact of palliative care on policy.
- The provision of a substantial number of training and education initiatives by a range of organisations.
- Existence of a national palliative care association.

Key figures like Dr Zipporah Ali have been active in the development of palliative care within Kenya and more widely in Africa. It is also very important to recognise the support of the Kenyan Ministry of Health, which has provided financial support and recognised palliative care as a central feature of health policy. Another major contributory factor has been the Kenya Hospices and Palliative Care Association

(KEHPCA), the national body that has represented all hospice and palliative care providers in Kenya since 2005. With government support, palliative care is now integrated into over 40 government hospitals, reaching out to all regions of the country, and palliative care is recognised as a patient's right. The Kenya National Patients' Rights Charter (Ministry of Health, 2013) recognises that the right to access health care includes: promotive, preventive, curative, reproductive, rehabilitative, and palliative care. Sheila Payne, quoted in Economist (2015, p. 13), states: "There's a general trend in which we're moving from the pioneer stage in many countries to people seeing how they can embed palliative care in healthcare systems. That's really important because that's about sustainability." Overall, this shows a successful model of collaboration at a national and international level.

KENYA: THE DEVELOPMENT OF PALLIATIVE CARE EDUCATION

Kenya has also seen an impressive development of palliative care education. This can be traced back to a collaboration between a Kenyan health institution, Nairobi Hospice, and a British educational institution, Oxford Brookes University, which started in 1992. This is outlined in Case study 3.

Case study 3: Collaboration between Kenya and UK to develop palliative care education

Nairobi Hospice was the first hospice to be opened in East Africa in 1990, offering services on an outpatient basis, in hospitals and in the patients' own homes within a 20 km radius, together with a weekly day-care service. Oxford Brookes University started offering the first Diploma of Higher Education in Palliative Care in the UK in 1991. In 1992, Brigid Sirengo, nurse and Chief Executive Officer of the Hospice, contacted the leader of the Oxford diploma course with a challenge to help the nurses, doctors, and other health care professionals who were working to develop palliative care in Africa. This sparked an initial visit to Nairobi in June 1992, and Brigid took the diploma, by correspondence, between 1993 and 1995.

The University decided to make a commitment to the international provision of palliative care education, and a formal agreement between the University and Nairobi Hospice was signed in June 2001, to teach the palliative care diploma in Nairobi. Teaching was delivered in Nairobi as three study blocks during an 18-month period, initially by "flying faculty". Since 2009, the course has been taught by the Nairobi Hospice team, as a University franchise.

The learning experience of students on the diploma is based on group-based classroom activities at the Nairobi Hospice, and on practice experience within the student's practice setting. The learning units or modules focus on: cultural and practical aspects of working with the dying, relationships with the dying and their families, symptom management and pain management, bereavement, and professional issues in palliative care.

Students develop skills in communication and relationships, critical appraisal and writing skills, skills in assessment and clinical management of patients, care of the dying and recently bereaved, conference participation and presentation, leadership, education, and management skills. Between study blocks, the student's learning is focused on their own practice.

The course team each have clinical and managerial responsibilities as well as education. However, education forms a central role within the hospice and each of them is involved in other teaching activities, mainly non-accredited courses and service mentorship schemes. As a result of Nairobi Hospice's pioneering role in Kenyan palliative care, the course team have been involved in key national and international conferences, national and international organisations (e.g. KEHPCA, African Palliative Care Association), and policy development with the Kenyan Ministry of Health.

The main countries that have sent students on the course are: Kenya, Malawi, Swaziland, Tanzania, Uganda, Zambia, and Zimbabwe, though there have also been students from Ethiopia, Sierra Leone, and the Gambia. The course is interprofessional, and most students have been nurses, doctors, and allied health professionals, with some social workers, counsellors, and chaplains. The course has developed a generation of pioneers and leaders in African palliative care. Students report that they are able to apply their new knowledge and skills directly in the care of the dying and their families. Alagie Omar Ceesay is a nurse working in the Gambia, who graduated in February 2014. He is a real pioneer of palliative care, initiating a service on his own and fighting to get it established: "I have just been promoted to Senior Nursing Officer two months ago. I am the focal Palliative Care expert in my hospital. The hospital is building an Anti-retro Viral (ART) Centre which is near completion and my boss has promised to make me the in-charge of the unit when initiated. I challenged my hospital that in order for palliative care to be effective, oral opioids especially liquid morphine must be available. Thank God this is now available and I feel more confident in dealing with my patients."

The development of the course can be viewed against the background of the internationalisation of higher education, and the increasing development of transnational education: education that crosses international borders (Altbach et al., 2009). Internationalisation of higher education may take the forms of students studying in another country, universities setting up a distant campus, or engaging in international partnerships. This has generally favoured the developed world, with its concentration of universities and supporting resources. In contrast, Sub-Saharan Africa has less well-developed educational capacity and infrastructure, with low rates of university enrolment: 5% of the age cohort compared to a global average of 26% (Altbach et al., 2009). Research and publication output is also amongst the lowest in the world (Bloom et al., 2006). An additional problem is the "brain drain" of African students who leave Africa to study, but do not return to make use of their education in their country of origin (Gyimah-Brempong et al., 2006).

The potential for growth of African institutions can be enhanced by the development of cross-border collaborations which give students in Africa access to the resources of universities in the developed world. These include existing curricula and learning materials, academic personnel, and e-libraries. Aside from these advantages, there are potential conflicts inherent in this sort of partnership. The transfer of curricula designed for the developed world may emphasise use of resources that are not freely available in Africa, and promote service models that do not fit readily into the African cultural context. However, there is evidence of service models in palliative care being successfully transferred and adapted to local conditions, and educational programmes can be modified to fit with African cultures. The experience in Nairobi shows that local personnel have the expertise to adapt learning materials, based on local knowledge and experience, even where literature on the African context is in short supply.

In education, KEHPCA has developed a National Training Curriculum in partnership with the Ministry of Health, to provide basic training for new palliative care professionals. Palliative care is now also included in both the Bachelor of Science in Nursing (BScN) curriculum (30 hours) and in the Kenya Registered Community Health Nursing (BASIC) curriculum (8 hours). Palliative care education is now well integrated into health care education, with mandatory palliative care education in all 5 medical schools and all 107 nursing schools (Rhee et al., 2017).

THE FUTURE: SUSTAINABILITY

Palliative care faces particular challenges of sustainability. It has traditionally been founded on charitable donations, ideally progressing to integration with mainstream health care. However, this process can be long and will only become well established when regular and reliable sources of income are available, ideally involving the country's own government.

Demand for palliative care education in Kenya and Sub-Saharan Africa is high and is likely to be so for many years to come. As the numbers of people needing palliative care increase, services continue to develop and to be supported by government health initiatives in some countries. The limiting factor for the growth of student numbers is funding. So far, the majority of Nairobi diploma students have been funded by charities. However, the world economy is in crisis and charitable funding can no longer be relied on to remain at sustainable levels. Economic factors are a major challenge for the future.

Sustainability in palliative care is not just about money, it also requires a suitable workforce, educated, supported, and maintained in the face of constant exposure to suffering and death. Ongoing specialist education and professional development is the key to sustaining the palliative care workforce (Cassel, 2012). For collaborations with palliative care in Africa to be sustainable, it is essential that developments are done in partnership, with a keen awareness of the African context of palliative care. Experts in the field warn against "parachute collaboration", where European partners drop in to teach or research; collaboration needs to involve a mutual and sustainable partnership (Radbruch & Brunsch-Radbruch, 2008). Indeed, the developed world also has much to learn from Africa, where a culture of inclusion and a focus on culturally appropriate and cost effective care provide an enviable model for the provision of services (Di Sorbo, 2011). Quoted in the Economist, Richard Harding describes how "African countries have succeeded in delivering high quality effective palliative care in the face of low resources and overwhelming need, and high- and middle-income countries would be wise to learn lessons from them".

International collaboration therefore has to be two-way: both partners need to make a long-term commitment to the development and maintenance of the programme, and to learning from each other.

KEY POINTS

- Palliative care services are expanding globally, and are present in some form in nearly 70% of the countries of the world, and this has been charted through several global surveys.
- International collaborations are the basis for many of the developments in palliative care services, education, and research.
- Palliative care development within countries is helped by local activism, community awareness, the availability of analgesia, education, and policy development, as well as international partnerships.
- Specific cases illustrate the processes and value of international partnerships in developing palliative care practice and education.
- For palliative care services to continue to develop globally, sustainable models need to be developed and adapted to changing circumstances.

REFERENCES

Altbach, PG, Reisberg, L, Rumbley, LE (2009) *Trends in Global Higher Education: Tracking an Academic Revolution.* A Report Prepared for the UNESCO 2009 World Conference on Higher Education. United Nations Educational, Scientific and Cultural Organization (UNESCO), Paris.

Bloom, D, Canning, D, Chan, K (2006) *Higher education and economic development in Africa.* Harvard University, Cambridge, MA.

Cassel, JB (2012) The importance of following the money in the development and sustainability of palliative care. *Palliative Medicine,* 27(2), 103–104.

Cleary, J, Radbruch, L, Torode, J, Cherny, NI (2013) Formulary availability and regulatory barriers to accessibility of opioids for cancer pain in Asia: a report from the Global Opioid Policy Initiative (GOPI). *Annals of Oncology,* (24)suppl_11, xi24–xi32. doi: 10.1093/annonc/mdt500

De Lima, L, Hanzah, E (2004) Socioeconomic, cultural and political issues in Palliative Care. In Bruera, E, De Lima, L, Wenk, R, Farr, W (eds.) *Palliative care in the developing world. Principles & practice.* International Association for Hospice & Palliative Care, Houston, pp. 23–37.

Di Sorbo, PG (2011) What Africa has to teach the United States about hospice and palliative care. *Journal of Palliative Care,* 14(2), 129–131.

The Economist Intelligence Unit (2015) *The 2015 quality of death index. Ranking palliative care across the world.* The Economist Intelligence Unit Limited, London.

Green, L (2019) Reflections on compassion in end of life care. https://lmiddletongreen .wordpress.com/

Gyimah-Brempong, K, Paddison, O, Mitiku, W (2006) Higher education and economic growth in Africa. *Journal of Development Studies*, 42(3), 509–529.

Harding, R, Higginson, IJ (2005) Palliative care in sub-saharan Africa. *Lancet*, 365, 1971–1977.

Lynch, T, Connor, S, Clark, D (2013) Mapping levels of palliative care development: a global update. *Journal of Pain and Symptom Management*, 45(6), 1094–1106.

Ministry of Health, Republic of Kenya (2013) *The Kenya national patients' rights charter.* http://medicalboard.co.ke/resources/PATIENTS_CHARTER_2013.pdf

Ministry of Health, Republic of Kenya (2015) *Kenya national strategy for the prevention and control of non-communicable diseases, 2015–2020.* https://www.who.int/nmh/ncd-task -force/kenya-strategy-ncds-2015-2020.pdf

Pav, S, Penfold, R, Watts, JH (2015) Palliative care in Cambodia: embryonic service provision and cultural barriers. *European Journal of Palliative Care*, 22(4), 202–204.

Radbruch, L, Brunsch-Radbruch, A (2008) Making it real: advances in palliative care in Africa. *European Journal of Palliative Care*, 15(1), 34–37.

Rhee, JY, Luyirika, E, Namisango, E, Powell, RA, Garralda, E, Pons, JJ, de Lima, L, Centeno, C (2017) *APCA atlas of palliative care in Africa.* IAHPC Press, Houston, TX.

Stjernswärd, J (2007) Palliative care: the public health strategy. *Journal of Public Health Policy*, 28, 42–55.

World Health Organisation (WHO) (2002) *WHO definition of palliative care.* https://www .who.int/cancer/palliative/definition/en/

Worldwide Hospice Palliative Care Alliance (2020) *Global Atlas of palliative care.* 2nd edn. Worldwide Hospice Palliative Care Alliance, London.

Wright, M, Wood, J, Lynch, T, Clark, D (2008) Mapping levels of palliative care development: a global view. *Journal of Pain & Symptom Management*, 35(5), 469–485. doi: 10.1016/j. jpainsymman.2007.06.006. Epub 2008 February 4.

CHAPTER 10

The future

Developing collaborative palliative care

....

Dave Roberts

OUTLINE

Collaborative practice is the norm in palliative care, based in an interprofessional, patient- and family-centred approach. There is a well-established culture of interprofessional working that has transferred across international boundaries. However, competing pressures on palliative and end of life care services may challenge this as we move into the future. These pressures include professional rivalry and competition, pressure to deliver value for money, and the dilution of services as palliative care reaches out into new settings. There is also a trend towards the deprofessionalisation of palliative care services that may either enhance or detract from collaborative working practices. New challenges to the provision of palliative care are also emerging with an ageing population, changing care settings, and viral pandemics. Palliative care will need to be robust and resilient to maintain its prominent place in health care, developing new models of care to meet demand.

WHAT WILL FUTURE PALLIATIVE AND END OF LIFE CARE LOOK LIKE?

As we move forward in the 21st century, there will be shifts in the ways that palliative care is practiced, in response to changing circumstances. Palliative care has already extended its reach, beyond its initial focus on cancer, to a range of long term conditions, and to end of life care in all settings, and whatever the cause.

The number of deaths per year in England and Wales are projected to increase and the average age of those dying will rise: by 2040, there will be 25% more deaths (Etkind et al., 2017), and 54% of people dying will be over 85 years, compared to 39% in 2014 (Bone et al., 2018). The place of death is also changing and will continue to do so. Hospices account for low numbers of deaths: roughly 5%, whereas

DOI: 10.4324/9781351113472-10

hospitals have, until recently, been the main place of death. Between 2004–2006, hospital deaths ran at around 58%, before falling below 50% in 2012 (Bone et al., 2018). This trend is likely to continue, with a higher proportion of deaths occurring in the patient's home, or in long term care facilities (care homes and nursing homes), assuming that long term care capacity rises in response to demand. If this is the case, then care and nursing homes will become an increasingly significant setting for end of life care.

Another major factor to consider is the complexity of care of an increasingly older population. With frailty and multiple comorbidity increasing, the demand for palliative care will increase as the population needs more specialist interventions and care staff need greater specialist support. Demand will rise at a higher rate than the death rate, increasing by as much 42% by 2040 (Etkind et al., 2017). Increased demand will be associated with new patterns of illness and dying, with multiple co-morbidities and long term conditions, and increasing incidence of cancer and dementia (see Chapter 3, case study 1 - Heart failure and end of life care, the *Better Together* project). A third of the population will die with dementia by 2050 (Calanzani et al., 2013). In addition to new challenges in long term care, the COVID-19 crisis has given rise to a new need for rapid palliative care response to an acute health emergency. This is likely to happen again, and palliative care services need to be involved in planning alongside colleagues based in acute hospital and community services.

Globally, the picture is different in countries with low and middle income economies. These countries represent the highest need for palliative care, but the lowest provision (O'Connor & Bermedo, 2014). Some of these are also facing the trend towards an older population with long term conditions as infectious diseases are brought increasingly under control. However, as we discussed in Chapter 9, the availability and utilisation of resources may be profoundly different. Many countries will not have enough trained palliative care staff, so education of this first line workforce is a high priority. Financing this, and the provision of basic services, requires advocacy and policy involvement at government level. Public attitudes in these countries also need to change to support a shift from curative to palliative services, to provide the most effective models for care delivery (Clark et al., 2018).

The future development of palliative care should continue to favour an interprofessional approach and collaboration between formal and informal service providers, as explored in Chapter 6. More broadly, this approach should include patient and public involvement in service evaluation and provision, and community and empowerment models of end of life care. The development of telemedicine or telehealth, and remote support (see Chapter 2) provides challenges and opportunities for professional services to adapt and review the nature of their role in palliative and end of life care. This has become an urgent issue to address as a new age of novel virus pandemics threatens existing patterns of social and professional interaction. The emergence of the COVID-19 crisis, ongoing at the time of writing, and bringing new challenges as we saw in Chapter 3, has resulted in unprecedented levels of enforced quarantine and social isolation. This has presented an impetus for the palliative care approach to be provided by remote consultation. The use of social media provides opportunities for professional groups to share information rapidly, provide informal means of professional and interprofessional development, and decrease social and professional isolation (McLoughlin et al., 2018).

WHAT PALLIATIVE CARE WORKFORCE WILL WE NEED?

The workforce of the future will continue to need palliative care specialists, generalists applying the palliative care approach, and informal care workers and carers with palliative care support. The hospice was the origin of the modern palliative care movement, and it retains a central place in the provision of palliative care. Whether it will continue to do so remains open to debate. Hospices usually provide specialist inpatient symptom management, psychosocial support, and care of the dying. They also function as centres of excellence in palliative care and a base for outreach and dissemination of good practice. However, they have their limitations. They have tended to be funded, at least initially, by charities, and this means they are less likely to be located in financially deprived areas. They have a patchy record of providing care to disadvantaged and minority groups. There is a limited evidence base for their effectiveness as a discrete service model (Calanzani et al., 2013).

As numbers requiring palliative care increase, and the setting of care moves substantially to the patient's home or to long term care, will there still be a place for the hospice, and what will it be? There will continue to be a need for a base for specialist expertise, including, for example, palliative care physicians, coordinating care and transitions between services, particularly through the work of community palliative care nurses, and supporting families, whether with the practical aspects of care, or social workers supporting family relationships and integrity. New models of care may be necessary, including hospice-supported beds in other settings and halfway house models which share elements of hospice and home care (Calanzani et al., 2013). Future hospice services must be flexible in response to complex and changing needs, engaging actively with community and long term care settings, and one model for achieving this, "InSup-C", was discussed in Chapter 2. It will also be essential to respond to the specific needs of individual patients, families, and communities, to ensure that services are inclusive and reach out to all members of society, as we saw in Chapter 4. However, none of this will be sustainable in the longer term without a clear evidence base and case for cost effectiveness.

Long term care settings are becoming a major location for the care of people with long term conditions, including cancer and dementia. Many people spend the last years of their lives in long term care facilities, so they may be both a home and a place of specialist care. They aim to maintain quality of life, enhancing the meaning of the individual's life and providing a meaningful death, as far as this is possible. They are also becoming the most common place of death in the UK. The future development of palliative care must, therefore, prioritise them. However, there are challenges in providing a consistent high standard of palliative and end of life care in long term facilities. Care homes are heavily regulated and this may make it harder for them to respond to changing demands and increasing complexity of their client group. Acute illness will frequently result in a hospital admission, and disrupt continuity of patient-centred care (Kaasalainen, 2020). If this is combined with high staff turnover and inadequate resources for staff education, it may prove difficult to develop and maintain a skilled workforce (Collingridge Moore et al., 2020). Some of the novel approaches to managing these challenges, including *Rapid Discharge Planning* and *Managed Clinical Networks*, are discussed in Chapters 2 and 3.

The family, however that is defined by its members, is the basic unit of palliative care, i.e. family-centred care, a theme explored particularly in Chapters 3, 4, and 5. Those who provide informal care at home are often called carers, though this is not often a term they would use themselves, preferring wife, mother, son, or friend, for example. The Macmillan/Ipsos Mori survey (2011) study of cancer carers suggests that 15% of the UK population have given some unpaid, informal support to a person with cancer in the last 12 months, and that 5% are currently doing this. They give an average of 15 hours of support a week, mostly emotional support (81%), but also errands like shopping or collecting prescriptions (51%), and taking or accompanying on visits or appointments (49%). 81% are affected in some way by the care they provide, involving emotional, social, occupational, and financial impacts. Only 45% get some form of support with their role. This is a substantial body of unpaid work. However, the work of informal caring is increasingly involving aspects of care that might have previously been seen as the realm of the professional. This includes watching for treatment side effects, helping manage pain, nausea or fatigue, administering medicine, deciding whether to call a doctor or administer medication, or changing bandages (Van Ryn et al., 2011). Following the death of the patient, carers often enter palliative care as clients of bereavement services. The carer is therefore at different times client, part of the unit of care, and collaborator.

However, the collaborative relationship with the carer in palliative care has not been fully developed. There have been numerous policy commitments to the involvement of service users or consumers (which would include both patients and their carers) in palliative care service planning, implementation, delivery, and evaluation, but there is limited evidence that this has translated into practice (Scholtz et al., 2019). In some ways this is surprising, given the commitment within palliative care services to patient- and family-centred care. However, service user involvement has similar problems to research in the field of palliative care: service users are at their most vulnerable when they are using the service. There is potential for greater involvement of service users in a meaningful collaboration to improve services, including palliative care education and research, if they are treated as equal partners and valued for their unique contribution (Scholtz et al., 2019).

WHAT ARE THE WORKFORCE EDUCATIONAL NEEDS?

Palliative care is provided by a range of different health and social care workers in a range of different settings (Table 1). They will require different levels of education and to support this, overall standards of competence for generalists and those using the palliative care approach have been developed by the European Association for

Palliative Care (Gamondi et al., 2013). These recognise the diverse and interprofessional nature of the palliative care workforce. As an international discipline, palliative care aims and principles are transferable not only across professional boundaries but also international ones, though the competencies have been developed for Europe (Gamondi et al., 2013) [see Box 10.1].

BOX 10.1 CORE INTERDISCIPLINARY COMPETENCIES IN PALLIATIVE CARE

The core interdisciplinary competencies promoted by the EAPC are:

1. Apply the core constituents of palliative care in the setting where patients and families are based.
2. Enhance physical comfort throughout patients' disease trajectories.
3. Meet patients' psychological needs.
4. Meet patients' social needs.
5. Meet patients' spiritual needs.
6. Respond to the needs of family carers in relation to short-, medium-, and long-term patient care goals.
7. Respond to the challenges of clinical and ethical decision-making in palliative care.
8. Practise comprehensive care co-ordination and interdisciplinary teamwork across all settings where palliative care is offered.
9. Develop interpersonal and communication skills appropriate to palliative care.
10. Practise self-awareness and undergo continuing professional development.

(Gamondi et al., 2013)

These are not an educational curriculum, rather they can be seen "as a means to share a common language for palliative care practice and education in Europe". It is suggested that optimal learning, for both specialist and generalist, is through interprofessional education, involving an interprofessional team of educators, though this can be difficult to achieve in practice, particularly in non-specialist areas (Gamondi et al., 2013).

Long term care settings in the developed world continue to see growing numbers of older people with complex care needs, including dementia, with its fluctuating patterns of frailty and cognitive impairment. Care homes have a mixture of registered nurses and care assistants, and they provide general basic palliative care to the dying and those with long term conditions. They will therefore benefit from educational programmes and other interventions that focus on improving the quality of care that they provide. Interventions may be delivered at different levels with different aims, in a similar way to the levels of psychological support discussed in Chapter 7. At an individual level, staff can be supported with the tools and skills for assessment, education, communication, and leadership. Groups or teams of staff can be supported with interprofessional education and clinical rounds, and at an organisational level interventions can focus on shared working with hospices and specialist palliative care teams, and also specialist palliative care units where these are established in care homes (Reitinger et al., 2013).

One such programme is PACE (PAlliative Care for Elderly people in long-term care facilities in Europe), which aims to train all staff within a facility to deliver basic general palliative care (Payne et al., 2019). The information pack emphasises the need for internal facilitation (1–3 key internal facilitators), and 6 steps of the programme (see Box 10.2). Each step involves the use of specific tools to support the intervention, recognising barriers and finding solutions, and training sessions.

BOX 10.2 PACE: 6 STEPS TO SUCCESS

Step 1: Discussions towards the end of life, gaining confidence in discussing future care and advance care planning.

Step 2: Assessment and review, recognising clinical signs as the patient approaches death and planning care accordingly.

Step 3: Co-ordination of palliative care, effective team work with regular interdisciplinary review meeting.

Step 4: Delivery of high quality palliative care: symptom control – pain, focusing on pain assessment and management as a major symptom.

Step 5: Care in the last days of life and the process of dying, recognising and responding when a resident is dying.

Step 6: Care after death, following good practices for the care of the body, and supporting family and friends.

(Payne et al., 2019)

For change to be effective, interventions should be more than simply training in order to achieve sustainability. PACE aims to develop a palliative care culture, i.e. embedding the palliative care approach within a facility (Reitinger et al., 2013). In order to achieve this, three strategic stages of implementation are necessary: establishing conditions to introduce the intervention, embedding the intervention within day-to-day practice, and sustaining ongoing change (Collingridge Moore et al., 2020). The success of interventions is very much dependent on the context, including, for example, the quality of communications within the facility.

NEW CHALLENGES IN THE ERA OF VIRAL PANDEMICS

The COVID-19 pandemic which emerged in 2019 has brought new challenges in the form of a surge of large numbers of acutely ill people with life-threatening illness.

Resources are stretched to and beyond their limits, services are overwhelmed, and countries across the globe are facing the most severe social restrictions in generations. Society is seeing mass mortality on a scale not usually seen outside of wars, or previous global pandemics like the Spanish Flu of a century ago.

This has brought demands on palliative care personnel, not necessarily new, in that these are with existing hospital and community based services, but novel in their scale and acuity. Those most at risk in the pandemic are the elderly and frail, including those who have long term illness and comorbidities. These are therefore, a familiar population to the palliative care specialist. The virus also brings familiar problems: facing uncertainty and death, end of life conversations, supporting the patient and family and their wishes through advance directives, and ensuring comfort and dignity at the time of dying. Palliative care specialists can therefore provide support and guidance to colleagues in acute services and primary care. The SWAN Model of Care described in Chapter 3 is a good example of this. Particular challenges arise where pressure on resources necessitate difficult discussions, for example, whether to admit to intensive care facilities, and it is here that palliative care expertise in complex decision-making and communication with the patient and their carers can be of greatest value (Lawrie & Murphy, 2020).

In addition, there is a role for palliative care in the strategic planning and management of viral pandemics. Downar & Seccarecci (2010) draw on a model for coping with "surge" capacity in intensive care, to propose a "palliative care pandemic plan" with four elements, "stuff, staff, space, and systems" (see Box 10.3).

BOX 10.3 PALLIATIVE CARE PANDEMIC PLAN

"Stuff" – a stockpile of necessary medication and equipment.

"Staff" – a core of palliative care specialists (doctors and nurses), education for frontline staff, standardised protocols for symptom management and end of life care, and specialist AHPs, social workers, and spiritual care staff to provide psychosocial and bereavement support.

"Space" – availability of wards and nonclinical areas to accommodate dying patients, and make good use of existing palliative care locations.

"Systems" – triage system for access to specialist palliative care services, direct consultation for non-specialist staff, including remote communication, and support for advance care plans.

(Downar & Seccarecci, 2010)

Clark et al., (2020) support this model, and emphasise the need for alternative facilities to cope with the surge in demand and the importance of psychosocial care, for patients and carers and also for staff. Patients may experience isolation and vulnerability and loss of family contacts. Staff will also have problems with stress, multiple mortalities, and fears for their own safety. Hospice and palliative care services can support the response to pandemics by flexible use of resources, and redeploying them, including volunteers, to the areas of greatest demand, being involved in triage and developing protocols for symptom management and psychological support, and training non-specialists in their use (Etkind et al., 2020). Arya et al. (2020) also raise the importance of working across diverse settings, including intensive care units, hospital wards, emergency departments, and long-term care, shared decision-making between clinicians and patients, including where this is severely restricted as a result of public health directives and resource availability. They also highlight the problems of how best to triage patients requiring palliative care, including how to manage those who are not offered life-sustaining measures.

Some of the most vulnerable at times of pandemics are those who live on the margins of society. They will find it harder to maintain a safe personal space, and access regular sources of food, shelter, and health care, with severe disruption to their support systems. Professionals engaged with them should take account of their needs for realistic public health guidance, managing their health including where necessary substance misuse, awareness of past trauma and its effects and support with advance care planning (Donald & Stajduhar, 2020).

INFORMAL GROUPS AND COMPASSIONATE COMMUNITIES

Whilst the focus of collaboration in palliative care is often on interprofessional practice, much of the actual care given to people with long term, life-threatening illness and at the end of life is informal, unpaid care. This is given by family, friends, and other members of their local community. Care after death in the form of bereavement care is largely provided by voluntary organisations and individual volunteers, on top of that given by family and friends. We know that the provision of palliative care is inconsistent, often driven initially by charities, and that this can further disadvantage deprived communities. Also, the professional basis of palliative care has been critiqued for its reliance on the traditional medical model (Morris & McDaid, 2017).

Challenging the professionalisation of dying, the emergence of social isolation as a health problem, and inequity of access to services has led to renewed interest in the public health approach to palliative care. Community programmes based on these principles can have a positive impact on social isolation, carer support, personal and community capacity, and wellbeing (Sallnow et al., 2016). Communities as a whole, therefore, have the capacity and responsibility to support the process of dying and its aftermath, a theme explored in Chapter 8.

The public health approach is the basis for the development of the Compassionate Community movement, one that has had an impact on informal groups like the Dying Matters Coalition in the UK. With the aim of helping people talk more openly about dying, death, and bereavement, and to make plans for the end of life, it shares the same principles as mainstream, professional palliative care, but adopts less formal community approaches. These can include quiz evenings about death and dying, local debates about helping disadvantaged communities, open days with funeral directors, crematoria, and hospices, or an art exhibition around dying and bereavement (Potter, n.d.). Although this approach signals a departure from the professionalisation of dying and death, it involves professionals, including primary and palliative care services. It therefore marks a point of collaboration between the community, informal agencies and volunteers, and professionals, though it is driven by voluntary agencies and community needs.

Interest in these informal groups is likely to grow. They can fill in some of the gaps left by professional services, like social isolation, they provide an opportunity for bereaved people to give something back, and they build social capital and wellbeing. They also provide a community focus for dealing with the real questions we all have about our mortality. It is notable that interest has grown in death cafes, an opportunity for people to meet and talk about death and dying with light refreshment, in response to the global COVID-19 pandemic (Brooks, 2020). These are clearly meeting a need that is not met by professional palliative care services. There is further scope within the public health model to develop palliative care based on a collaboration between specialist and generalist palliative care services, local communities, and the broader civic sectors of society (Abel et al., 2018).

The last word goes to the authors of a paper on community action.

> Previous experiences have shown that implementation of these kinds of initiatives are highly context-dependent and their success requires a deep understanding of the dynamics and networks of care, and the needs and aspirations of people and caregivers at the end of life.
>
> Communities matter! Their culture, values, identities shape the way they approach dying.
>
> *(Hasson et al., 2018)*

KEY POINTS

- Collaboration is the working model on which palliative care was founded, and it is the way forward for its further development.
- A collaborative approach has been evident at each stage of the growth of palliative care out of its original hospice base: collaborations within hospitals, primary care, and the community.
- Palliative care is now moving into new areas of practice, and this has been particularly striking during the emergence of new viral pandemics.
- Further opportunities can be developed with community groups, recognising that the community is the natural place for death, dying, and bereavement.
- As these develop, it will be important to work with an awareness of local contexts and the complexity of working across professional and cultural boundaries.

REFERENCES

Abel, J, Kelleher, A, Karapliagou, A (2018) Palliative care—the new essentials. *Annals of Palliative Medicine*, 7(S2), S3–14. doi: 10.21037/apm.2018.03.04

Arya, A, Buchman, S, Gagnon, B, Downar, J (2020) Pandemic palliative care: beyond ventilators and saving lives. *CMAJ*, 192, E400–E404. doi: 10.1503/cmaj.200465; early-released March 31, 2020.

Bone, A, Gomes, B, Etkind, S, Verne, J, Murtagh, F, Evans, C, Higginson, I (2018) What is the impact of population ageing on the future provision of end-of-life care? Population-based projections of place of death. *Palliative Medicine*, 32(2), 329–336. doi: 10.1177/0269216317734435

Brooks, L (2020) Death cafes see surge of interest in online events. The global movement encourages honest and open conversation about mortality. *The Guardian*, 13 April 2020. https://www.theguardian.com/society/2020/apr/13/death-cafes-see-surge-of-interest-in-online-events

Calanzani, N, Higginson, IJ, Gomes, B (2013) *Current and future needs for hospice care: an evidence based report*. Cicely Saunders International, Kings College London. http://www.helpthehospices.org.uk/commission

Clark, D, Krawzyck, M, Richards, N, Whitelaw, S, Bell, A (2020) *Palliative care and Covid-19*. 19 March 2020. University of Glasgow End of Life Studies Group. http://endoflifestudies.academicblogs.co.uk/palliative-care-and-covid-19/

Clark, J, Barnes, A, Gardiner, C (2018) Re-framing global palliative care advocacy for the sustainable development goal era: a qualitative study of the views of international palliative care experts. *Journal of Pain and Symptom Management*, 56(3), 363–370.

Collingridge Moore, D, Payne, S, Van den Block, L, Ling, J, Froggatt, K (2020) Strategies for the implementation of palliative care education and organizational interventions in long-term care facilities: a scoping review. *Palliative Medicine*, 34(5), 558–570. doi: 10.1177/0269216319893635

Donald, E, Stajduhar, K (2020) COVID-19: equity-informed palliative care & social disadvantage. ePac 30 March 2020. https://www.equityinpalliativecare.com/post/covid-19-equity-informed-palliative-care-and-social-disadvantage

Downar, J, Seccareccia, D (2010) Palliating a pandemic: 'all patients must be cared for'. *Journal of Pain and Symptom Management*, 39(2), 291–295. doi: 10.1016/j.jpainsymman.2009.11.241

Etkind, SN, Bone, AE, Gomes, B, Lovell, N, Evans, C, Higginson, I, Murtagh, F (2017) How many people will need palliative care in 2040? Past trends, future projections and implications for services. *BMC Medicine*, 15, 102.

Etkind, SN, Bone, AE, Lovell, N, Cripps, RL, Harding, R, Higginson, IJ, Sleeman, KE (2020) The role and response of palliative care and hospice services in epidemics and pandemics: a rapid review to inform practice during the COVID-19 pandemic. *Journal of Pain and Symptom Management*, 60(1), e31–e40. doi: 10.1016/j.jpainsymman.2020.03.029

Gamondi, C, Larkin, P, Payne, S (2013) Core competencies in palliative care: an EAPC White Paper on palliative care education – part 1. *European Journal of Palliative Care*, 20(2), 86–91.

Hasson, N, Grajales, M, Grajales, I, Espiau, G, Nuño, R, Urtaran, M (2018) Building a narrative for compassionate communities: the case of Getxo Zurekin. *International Journal of Integrated Care*, 18(S2), A321, 1–8. doi: 10.5334/ijic.s2321

Kaasalainen, S (2020) Current issues with implementing a palliative approach in long-term care: where do we go from here? *Palliative Medicine*, 34(5), 555–557. doi: 10.1177/0269216320916118

Lawrie, I, Murphy, F (2020) *COVID-19 and palliative, end of life and bereavement care in secondary care role of the specialty and guidance to aid care*. The Northern Care Alliance

NHS Group and the Association for Palliative Medicine of Great Britain and Ireland. https://apmonline.org/wp-content/uploads/2020/03/COVID-19-and-Palliative-End-of-Life-and-Bereavement-Care-22-March-2020.pdf

Macmillan/Ipsos Mori (2011) *More than a million.* Macmillan, Ipso Mori, London.

McLoughlin, C, Patel, K, O'Callaghan, T, Reeves, S (2018) The use of virtual communities of practice to improve interprofessional collaboration and education: findings from an integrated review. *Journal of Interprofessional Care,* 32(2), 136–142.

Morris, L, McDaid, M (2017) Compassionate communities - from frailty to community resilience – making a public health approach to end of life care a reality. *International Journal of Integrated Care,* 17(5), A134, 1–8. doi: 10.5334/ijic.3442

O'Connor, SR, Bermedo, MCS (2014) *Global atlas of palliative care at the end of life.* World Health Organization, Worldwide Palliative Care Alliance, Geneva. https://www.who.int/nmh/Global_Atlas_of_Palliative_Care.pdf

Payne, S, Froggatt, K, Hockley, J, Sowerby, E, Collingridge Moore, D, Kylänen, M, Oosterveld-Vlug, M, Pautex, S, Szczerbińska, K, Van Den Noortgate, N, Van den Block, L (2019) *PACE steps to success programme. Steps towards achieving high quality palliative care in your care home.* Vrije Universiteit Brussel (VUB), End-of-Life Care Research Group.

Potter, L. Why should we develop compassionate communities? *Dying Matters.* https://www.dyingmatters.org/sites/default/files/user/documents/Resources/Community%20Pack/1-Introduction-1.pdf

Reitinger, E, Froggatt, K, Brazil, K, Heimerl, K, Hockley, J, Kunz, R, Morbey, H, Parker, D, Husebo, B, Reitinger, E, et al. (2013) Palliative care in long-term care settings for older people: findings from an EAPC Taskforce. *European Journal of Palliative Care,* 20(5), 251–253.

Sallnow, L, Khan, F, Uddin, N, Kellehear, A (2016) The impact of a new public health approach to end-of-life care: a systematic review. *Palliative Medicine,* 30(3), 200–211. doi: 10.1586/erp.11.18

Scholz, B, Bevan, A, Georgousopoulou, E, Collier, A, Mitchell, I (2019) Consumer and carer leadership in palliative care academia and practice: a systematic review with narrative synthesis. *Palliative Medicine,* 33(8), 959–968. doi: 10.1177/0269216319854012

van Ryn, M, Sanders, S, Kahn, K, van Houtven, C, Griffin, JM, Martin, M, Atienza, AA, Phelan, S, Finstad, D, Rowland, J (2011) Objective burden, resources, and other stressors among informal cancer caregivers: a hidden quality issue? *Psycho-Oncology,* 20, 44–52.

Index

activity scheduling 79
acute care model 3–4, 34; ideology of rescue 18
acute myeloid leukaemia 41
administration of injectable medication: in a community services setting 46; home-based care and 44
Advance care planning 18, 43, 44, 115, 117; advance directives 116
advocacy 103, 111
Africa: palliative care education in 105–107; sustainability of palliative care in 107–108
African-Caribbean community: bereavement 89; death rituals 87–88; end of life care in 86–87, 88; loss and 91; resilience in 89; slavery and 87–88; structural inequality and 90; see also minorities
African Palliative Care Association (APCA) 103
Ambitions for Palliative and End of Life Care 84
anxiety: interventions 76; management 76, 77; symptoms 75–76; triggers 75
assessment 115; of depression 78
availability of resources 16, 17

bereavement 44, 50, 51, 55, 57, 65, 77–78, 86, 88, 113; culture and 89; stoicism and 87; SWAN team 34
"Better Together project 33
blood transfusions, home-based care and 42
boundaries 26, 27, 32; family 51

breast cancer 53, 78–79; see also cancer
Bridges 65; care coordinators 61–62; childcare 63–64

Cambodia 99, 101
cancer 13–14, 41, 42, 43, 53, 54, 55, 60, 63, 64, 70, 73, 74, 75, 113; anxiety and 76–77; depression and 78–79
Care and Quality Commission 40
care coordinators 61–62, 63, 64, 65
care homes 16, 112–113, 114; end of life care and 17; see also home-based care; hospices
caregivers 84, 113; see also family(ies); nurses
chemotherapy 13, 41, 53
Childhood Bereavement Network 51–52
children 56, 63–64; family therapy and 51–52
chronic obstructive pulmonary disease (COPD) 17; symptom management 42–43
cognitive behaviour therapy (CBT) 76, 77, 79
collaboration 2, 3, 8, 9, 10, 12, 15, 18, 20, 26, 62, 110; with family members 49–50; inter-cultural 92–94; international 98, 99, 102, 105–107, 108; national 103; in non-malignant conditions 31–32; palliative care and 4–5; "parachute" 107–108; service level agreements 45–46; between service providers 10; systems theory and 49; transitioning from home to care home 17; see also integrated palliative care; interprofessional

practice (IPP); multidisciplinary team (MDT); partnerships; teamwork(ing); transitioning between care settings
community healthcare 59, 60, 73, 83, 117; African-Caribbean 87–88, 89; barriers to integrating team working 66, 67; Bridges service 61; Dying Matters Coalition 117–118; end of life care 13–14, 84–-85; frameworks 31; H@H 62; home-based blood transfusions 42; inter-cultural collaboration 92–94; leadership and 65–66; security and 46; women and 89
Compassion Fatigue Awareness Project 79
Compassionate Cities 9, 82, 83, 85; Charter 83; inter-cultural collaboration 92–94; volunteers 91–92; *see also* African-Caribbean community
consent 16
content of care 6, 13, 14–15
continuous subcutaneous infusion (CSCI) 14
coordination 3
coping 74, 87, 116; with anxiety 76; meaning-based 74; problem-based 74–75; problem-solving and 74–75
core palliative care team 6
COVID-19 pandemic 34, 91, 111, 115–116, 118
cultural factfile approach to end of life care 85
culture: bereavement and 89; end of life care and 85–86
curiosity, systemic thinking and 53
cygnets 34; *see also* SWAN team

data protection 16
death/dying 91–92; preferred place of 13, 39, 62, 63, 110–111, 112; professionalisation of 52, 117; rituals and 87, 88
dementia 19, 111, 114
demoralisation 78, 79; *see also* depression
depression 72; activity scheduling 79; cancer and 78–79; managing in palliative care 78–79; screening for 77–78; spectral model of 77; *see also* bereavement
distress 49, 52, 56–57, 70, 71, 72, 79; recognising and responding to 73; *see also* psychological care
Distress Thermometer 78
District Nurses 14, 17, 31, 43, 63, 73
Dying Matters Coalition 117–118
Dying Well in Custody Charter 46

education 113–114; Oxford diploma course 105, 106; "parachute collaboration" and 107–108
electronic patient records 16; Gold Line service 22

end of life care (EoLC) 2, 12–13, 14, 15, 18, 19, 20, 82–83; accessibility to 27, 39, 43; *Ambitions for Palliative and EoLC. A national framework for local action 2015–2020* 7–8; *Care for dying adults in the last days of life* 8; community engagement and 84–-85; culture and 85, 86; *End of Life Care Strategy* 7; *Gold Standards Framework* (GSF) 7; home-based care 39–40; hospitals and 13; inter-cultural collaboration 92–94; *Liverpool Care Pathway for the Dying Patient* (LCP) 7; *One Chance to Get it Right* 7; resuscitation 32; SWAN team 34; symptom management and 42–43; training 46
ensuring access to care 45
European Association for Palliative Care (EAPC) 2

family(ies) 9, 54, 82, 113, 117; bereavement 51; collaboration with 49–50; ecomaps 56; as informal caregivers 43–44; resilience 57; social care 70; SWAN team and 34; therapy 50; *see also* systemic practice
Fast Track *see* Rapid Discharge (RDP)
friends, as informal caregivers 43–44, 117

General Data Protection Regulation (GDPR) 16
general palliative care 1–2, 5
geriatric medicine 18
global palliative care 9–10, 98–99
Gold Standards Framework (GSF) 7, 31
GPs 31–32
grief 88, 90, 93; as a social relationship 86–87; *see also* bereavement; psychological care

"hard to reach" groups 40
heart failure 111; symptom management 42–43
HIV/AIDS 102
holistic care 1, 2, 4, 5, 16, 26, 27, 28, 30, 33, 40, 44, 45, 49, 51, 62, 69, 80, 82
Holistic Needs Assessment 73
home-based care 33, 38, 39; administration of injectable medication 44; based on individual need 41; establishing a ceiling of treatment 41; family/friends as informal caregivers 43–44; making the service fit the patient 39–40; symptom management and 42–43; "transfusion tether" and 42
Hospice at Home (H@H) 62, 66, 67; care coordinators 64–65; childcare 63–64

hospices 16, 17, 60, 85, 110–111, 112, 115; integrating with local healthcare 20, 21; Kenyan 103; *see also* home-based care

Hospital Anxiety and Depression Scale (HADS) 78

hospitals 13, 15; ideology 18; palliative care and 7, 14–15; palliative care units (PCUs) 103

ideology 17; of palliative care 18

inequality(ies) 9, 60, 87; access to palliative and end of life care 27, 39, 44–45, 86; in provision of end of life care 40; social capital and 83; structural 90

informal caregivers 43–44

information logistics 6, 15–16, 67

integrated care 3

integrated hospice services 20, 21

integrated palliative care 5–7, 8, 59, 66; availability of resources 16, 17; barriers to 66, 67; co-location 63; content of care 6, 13, 14–15; core team 6; H@H 62; information logistics 6, 15–16; key domains of care delivery 6; leadership and 65–66; patient flow 6, 15, 26; patient flow and 14–15; teamworking and 27; transitions and 12–13

Integrated Palliative Care in Cancer and Chronic Conditions (InSup-C) 21, 112

inter-cultural collaboration 92–94

international collaboration 98, 99, 102, 105–107, 108; *see also* Africa; Cambodia; Kenya

interprofessional education (IPE) 4

interprofessional practice (IPP) 2, 4, 8, 9, 82, 110, 111; "Better Together" project 33–34; core competencies 114; education 30–31; language and 32–33; for patients with non-malignant conditions 31–32; roles and 27, 30; supporting one another 30–31; *see also* multidisciplinary team (MDT)

interventions, psychological care 70–72, 73

Kenya: collaboration with United Kingdom 105–107; National Patients' Rights Charter 105; palliative care in 102–105

Kenya Hospices and Palliative Care Association (KEHPCA) 103, 104–105, 107

key worker role 31

Lancelot Oncology Commission 8

leadership, integrated palliative care and 65–66

Leadership Alliance for the Care of Dying People (LACDP), *One Chance to Get it Right* 7

LGBTQ+ community, accessibility to palliative and end of life care 44–45

Liverpool Care Pathway for the Dying Patient (LCP) 7

long-term oxygen therapy (LTOT) 17

loss 90–92

Managed Clinical Networks (MCNs) 22, 23

Marie Curie 8, 44, 45

mental health services, palliative care and 45–46

minorities 82, 86; access to palliative and end of life care 44–45, 85; racism and 88

multidisciplinary team (MDT) 2, 26, 27, 52, 70; "Better Together" project 33–34; boundaries 27, 32; core competencies 114; enhancing understanding of systemic perspectives and tools 56; family/friends as informal caregivers 43–44; H@H 63; home-based care and 39–40; joint reviews 43; meetings 2; for patients with non-malignant conditions 31–32; roles 27, 69; service level agreements 45–46; tiered approaches to assessment and management of distress 56–57

Murray Hall service partnership 60, 61, 62, 65, 66

National Health Service (NHS) 9, 27, 59, 60; *End of Life Care Strategy* 7

National Institute for Health and Care Excellence (NICE) 31; *Care for dying adults in the last days of life* 8; *End of Life Care for Adults: Service Delivery* 8; *Improving Supportive and Palliative Care for Adults with Cancer* 70; *Quality Standards* 8

National Palliative and End of Life Care Partnership 18; *Ambitions for Palliative and EoLC. A national framework for local action 2015–2020* 7–8

networks 3, 83, 84, 85

non-malignant conditions: clinical uncertainty of 32; collaborative palliative care 31–32

nurses 65, 70, 75; "Better Together" project 33; caring for patients with non-malignant conditions 31–32; clinical specialist 43; community 17; District 17; H@H 62; mental health specialist 79; palliative care education and 106; SWAN team 34

pain 2, 72; anxiety and 76; management 13–14; opioids and 101; "total" 51
palliative care 2, 3, 5, 18, 49, 82; "assumptions" and 45; in Cambodia 101; collaboration and 4, 4–5; community settings 5; core interdisciplinary competencies 114; COVID-19 and 111, 115–116; definition 2; depression and 78–79; deprofessionalisation of 110; education 105, 113–114; end of life care and 2; general 1–2; global 9–10, 98–99; "hard to reach" groups and 40; holistic approach 69; hospital settings 5; ideology of 18; increasing demand for 111; informal 117–118; integrated 5–7; inter-cultural collaboration 92–94; in Kenya 102–105; levels of development 104; long-term 112; opioids and 101; Oxford diploma course 105–106; pandemic plan 116–117; professionalisation of 84–85; psychological care 9; public health approach 9; service level agreements 45–46; social media and 111–112; specialist 1, 5, 16, 27, 43, 70, 112; sustainability and 107–108; systemic thinking and 50–52; teamworking in 27–28; training 46; trends 110–111; in underdeveloped countries 111; see also end of life care (EoLC); psychological care
PAlliative Care for Elderly people (PACE) 115
Palliative Care Public Health Strategy 98
pandemics 111; palliative care and 116–117; see also COVID-19 pandemic
"parachute collaboration" 107–108
Parkinson's disease 45
patient flow 6, 15, 26
patients, as team members 32
PEG feeding 19–20
pharmacies 43
posttraumatic stress disorder (PTSD) 74
poverty 83, 90
preferred place of death 13, 33, 39, 40, 46, 62
Primary Care Groups (PCGs) 59, 60
Primary Care Trusts (PCTs) 59
prions, as place of care 38–40, 46
problem-based coping 74–75
prognostication 15, 42
psychological care 9, 51, 69; anxiety and 75–77; coping 74, 75; demands of 79–80; depression and 77–78, 79; distress and 72–73; level 1 70–71; level 2 71; level 3 71; level 4 71–72; levels of 70; personal reactions 73–74; problem-solving 74–75; suffering and 72
psychosocial care 2, 15, 57, 69, 70
public health approach 9, 60, 83, 85, 118; see also community healthcare

racism 88, 93
Rapid Discharge (RDP) 20
referral systems 6
rehabilitation 18
residential care 13; see also care homes
resilience: community 85–86, 88; in the African-Caribbean community 88–89; family 9, 57; loss and 90; personal 74, 79, 90
resources 6
resuscitation 32
risk management 18
roles 3–5, 10, 18, 20, 23, 26–27, 30–32, 34, 42–44, 46, 50, 52–53, 61, 66, 69–70, 72, 77, 83–84, 86, 89, 91–93, 106, 111, 113; role conflict 9, 79–80; role-modelling 90
Royal College of Physicians 8

sadness 77; see also depression
Sandwell PCT 59–60, 66; Bridges service 61, 62; Hospice at Home (H@H) 62; see also Bridges; Hospice at Home (H@H)
Saunders, C. 1, 51
self-care 79–80
service level agreements 45–46
sexual orientation, and access to palliative and end of life care 44–45
"Six Steps to Success in End of Life Care" 31
slavery 87–88
social care 70
social death 87
social media, palliative care and 111–112
social work(ers) 30, 51
South Africa 104
specialist palliative care 1, 5, 16, 27, 43, 70, 112; H@H 62; teamworking and 30–31
spectral model of depression 77
stereotypes 87, 91
stoicism 87, 90
structural inequality 90
substance abuse 45
suffering 72, 73, 79, 92–93; see also psychological care
support at a distance 16
sustainability, palliative care and 107–108
SWAN team 34, 116
symptom management 46, 64–65; end of life care and 42–43
systemic practice 49, 57; assets-based philosophies and 57; circularity 53, 54–55; curiosity and 53; enhancing the MDT's understanding of systemic perspectives and tools 56; hypotheses 52–53; neutrality and 53; palliative care and 50–52; Post Milan approaches 50; tiered approaches to assessment and management of distress 56–57

teamwork(ing) 3, 26; challenges 28, 30; fragmentation and 27; key worker role 31; palliative care and 27–28; patients as team members 32; roles 27, 69; supporting one another 30–31
telemedicine 23, 111; Gold Line service 22
"total pain" 51
transitioning between care settings 39; curative to palliative care 13–15; home to care home 17; hospital to home 20; Managed Clinical Networks (MCNs) and 22, 23
trauma 57

Uganda 102, 104
United Kingdom 13, 20, 39; collaboration with Kenya 105–107; Data Protection Act (2018) 16

volunteers 2, 63, 84, 85, 117; Bridges service 61; Compassionate Cities 91–92; *see also* community healthcare

wider professional community 6, 7
women, communitarian work and 89, 92
World Health Organisation (WHO) 60, 103; Palliative Care Public Health Strategy 98

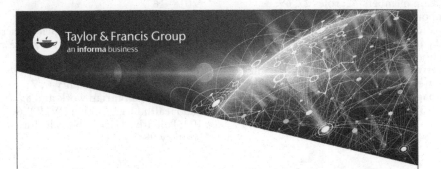

Printed in the United States
by Baker & Taylor Publisher Services

Printed in the United States
by Baker & Taylor Publisher Services